WEIGHT CONTROL

This new series is designed to meet the growing demand for current, accessible information about the increasingly popular wellness approach to personal health. The result of a collaborative effort by a highly professional writing, editorial, and publishing team, the *Wellness* series consists of 16 volumes, each on a single topic. Each volume in this attractively produced series combines original material with carefully selected readings, relevant statistical data, and illustrations. The series objectives are to increase awareness of the value of a wellness approach to personal health and to help the reader become a more informed consumer of health-related information. Employing a critical thinking approach, each volume includes a variety of assessment tools, discusses basic concepts, suggests key questions, and provides the reader with a list of resources for further exploration.

James K. Jackson	Wellness: AIDS, STD, & Other Communicable Diseases
Richard G. Schlaadt	Wellness: Alcohol Use & Abuse
Richard G. Schlaadt	Wellness: Drugs, Society, & Behavior
Robert E. Kime	Wellness: Environment & Health
Gary Klug & Janice Lettunich	Wellness: Exercise & Physical Fitness
James D. Porterfield & Richard St. Pierre	Wellness: Healthful Aging
Robert E. Kime	Wellness: The Informed Health Consumer
Paula F. Ciesielski	Wellness: Major Chronic Diseases
Robert E. Kime	Wellness: Mental Health
Judith S. Hurley	Wellness: Nutrition & Health
Robert E. Kime	Wellness: Pregnancy, Childbirth, & Parenting
David C. Lawson	Wellness: Safety & Accident Prevention
Randall R. Cottrell	Wellness: Stress Management
Richard G. Schlaadt	Wellness: Tobacco & Health
Randall R. Cottrell	Wellness: Weight Control
Judith S. Hurley & Richard G. Schlaadt	Wellness: The Wellness Life-Style

WEIGHT CONTROL

Randall R. Cottrell

WELLNESS

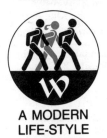

A MODERN
LIFE-STYLE
LIBRARY

The Dushkin Publishing Group, Inc./Sluice Dock, Guilford, CT 06437

AAZ2086

Library of Congress Catalog Card Number: 91-072191
Manufactured in the United States of America
First Edition, First Printing
ISBN: 0-87967-878-X

Library of Congress Cataloging-in-Publication Data

Cottrell, Randall R., Weight Control (Wellness)
     1. Obesity. 2. Reducing. 3. Body weight. I. Title. II. Series.
RC628   613.25   91-072191   ISBN 0-87967-878-X

Please see page 155 for credits.

The procedures and explanations given in this publication are based on research and consultation with medical and nursing authorities. To the best of our knowledge, these procedures and explanations reflect currently accepted medical practice; nevertheless, they cannot be considered absolute and universal recommendations. For individual application, treatment suggestions must be considered in light of the individual's health, subject to a doctor's specific recommendations. The authors and the publisher disclaim responsibility for any adverse effects resulting directly or indirectly from the suggested procedures, from any undetected errors, or from the reader's misunderstanding of the text.

RANDALL R. COTTRELL

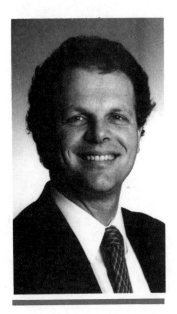

Randall Russell Cottrell was born in Oberlin, Ohio, in 1951. He is a graduate of Bowling Green State University, from which he received both a B.S. and an M.Ed., and the Pennsylvania State University, from which he received his doctorate in health education in 1982. He is currently Associate Professor and Head of the Department of Health and Nutrition Sciences at the University of Cincinnati. During the course of his professional career, Dr. Cottrell has written on a variety of health-related topics. In addition to his 2 titles in the *Wellness* series, Dr. Cottrell has published some 20 articles and is working on a text on worksite health promotion. As a speaker, he has addressed a diverse set of audiences including public school teachers, corporate executives, college students, mental patients, and Oregon forestry workers.

WELLNESS:
A Modern Life-Style Library

General Editors
Robert E. Kime, Ph.D.
Richard G. Schlaadt, Ed.D.

Authors
Paula F. Ciesielski, M.D.
Randall R. Cottrell, Ed.D.
Judith S. Hurley, M.S., R.D.
James K. Jackson, M.D.
Robert E. Kime, Ph.D.
Gary A. Klug, Ph.D.
David C. Lawson, Ph.D.
Janice Lettunich, M.S.
James D. Porterfield
Richard St. Pierre, Ph.D.
Richard G. Schlaadt, Ed.D.

Developmental Staff
Irving Rockwood, Program Manager
Paula Edelson, Series Editor
James D. Porterfield, Developmental Editor
Wendy Connal, Administrative Assistant
Jason J. Marchi, Editorial Assistant

Editing Staff
John S. L. Holland, Managing Editor
Elizabeth Jewell, Copy Editor
Diane Barker, Editorial Assistant
Mary L. Strieff, Art Editor
Robert Reynolds, Illustrator

Production and Design Staff
Brenda S. Filley, Production Manager
Whit Vye, Cover Design and Logo
Jeremiah B. Lighter, Text Design
Libra Ann Cusack, Typesetting Supervisor
Charles Vitelli, Designer
Meredith Scheld, Graphics Assistant
Steve Shumaker, Graphics Assistant
Lara M. Johnson, Graphics Assistant
Juliana Arbo, Typesetter
Richard Tietjen, Editorial Systems Analyst

THE PROBLEM OF WEIGHT MANAGEMENT has fascinated me for many years. As a child, I remember feeling that I was too fat. I always wore the "husky" size jeans and seemed somewhat bigger than my friends. Fortunately, around puberty I slimmed down and through regular exercise and dietary control have managed to maintain my weight in the acceptable range. This has not been easy, however. I have a voracious appetite for sweets and am constantly aware that someday I could again slip into the overweight category—or, more properly and as is discussed in the book, the overfat category.

In addition to my own weight problems, I have watched many of my friends and family members struggle with unwanted pounds. Inevitably, they tell me how much they want to lose weight, yet they cannot seem to succeed. They try diet program after diet program, and the scenario is nearly always the same. First, they identify a new "wonder diet" that has been recommended by a friend or has worked for some celebrity. Then there is a burst of hope and confidence as they start the program and the first few pounds actually disappear. Over the long run, however, the norm is failure. In some cases, the new regimen lasts only a few weeks before discouragement sets in, and the search for a new diet that will work resumes. In other cases, the original weight loss goal is achieved but cannot be maintained. Then I watch as slowly but surely the individual regains the lost pounds while feeling worse and worse about himself or herself in the process.

But there is a better way, as has been convincingly demonstrated by a number of my friends who have succeeded in their quest to lose weight. Invariably, this has been because they followed the principles set forth in the pages that follow. The basic elements of this strategy are simple—a lifelong change in dietary behavior coupled with a well-designed exercise program.

The book begins by examining the latest research on why people gain weight and why it is so difficult to lose. Next, it discusses the health problems associated with being overfat. Effective weight control is presented as the outcome of a permanent life-style change that involves behavior modification, diet, and exercise. Self-tests, readings, and practical guidelines are provided throughout, and a variety of additional resources are listed in the appendix.

This is not a definitive work, but rather a place to begin. The central objective of this book is not to make you into an instant expert but to help you learn to think critically about the information on weight control and health with which all of us are bombarded almost daily. Only then will you be able to distinguish weight control fact from weight control myth, and only then will you be an informed health consumer.

Numerous people have had a role in the development of this book. I would like ot thank Richard G. Schlaadt and Robert E. Kime of the University of Oregon for their role in initiating the process that led to the publication of the *Wellness* series and for their encouragement throughout. I would like to thank Irving Rockwood, Paula Edelson, Wendy Connal, and Jason J. Marchi of The Dushkin Publishing Group, and James D. Porterfield, the developmental editor, for their editorial assistance and continual guidance. A special thanks must go to Judy Simon of the University of Maryland for her careful review of the manuscript and many useful suggestions. And most important, I must thank my wife, Karen, and my sons, Kyle and Kory. They are my support system, my inspiration, and my joy.

Randall R. Cottrell
Cincinnati, OH

Contents

1

Weight Control: A Problem of Caloric Balance

Page 1

2

Factors Affecting Weight

Page 26

5

Fads, Gimmicks, Gadgets, and Quick Weight-Loss Programs

Page 95

6

Other Weight-Related Problems

Page 113

FIGURES

TABLES

Weight Control: A Problem of Caloric Balance

AMERICANS CONSUME MORE FAT per capita than any other nation in the world. They also consume more than 90 percent of the world's foods high in saturated fats and processed sugars. The result of these national preoccupations with food and effortless living is that an estimated 60 to 70 million adults and 10 to 12 million teenagers are "too fat" by a total of 2.3 billion pounds. In calories, this excess fat represents an energy equivalent of 5.7 trillion **kilocalories (kcal)** or the potential energy in 1.3 billion gallons of gasoline. This is sufficient energy to power 900,000 automobiles a year or provide the annual residential electrical requirements of Boston, Chicago, San Francisco, and Washington, DC. [1]

THE SCOPE OF THE PROBLEM: AN OVERVIEW

Obesity is one of the major health problems of our time. It is estimated that 34 million Americans are at least 20 percent above their optimum weight. [2] That is the point, experts agree, at which excess weight has an adverse effect on the health of the person carrying it. [3] Based on recent prevalence studies, the state of West Virginia held the dubious distinction of having the most overweight population. Twenty-four percent of all West Virginians were overweight. Other states with high overweight populations included Wisconsin (23 percent), North Dakota (23 percent), North Carolina (22 percent), Kentucky (22 percent), and Missouri (22 percent). Two states, Utah and Hawaii, tied for the honor of having the least overweight populations, with 14 percent each. [4]

Kilocalorie (kcal): The most widely used measure of the energy content of foods, a kilocalorie is defined as the amount of heat necessary to raise the temperature of one *kilogram* of water one degree Celsius at normal atmospheric pressure; commonly referred to as "calorie" and thus sometimes confused with the "small calorie" used in physics and chemistry; the latter equals the amount of heat necessary to raise the temperature of one *gram* of water by one degree Celsius at normal atmospheric pressure.

(continued on p. 4)

Battling the Bulge at an Early Age

Too many children carry the weight of the world on their shoulders—and around their middles. Today's youngsters are flabbier and increasingly unable to measure up to standard levels in tests of physical fitness. And they're likely to grow up as obese adults, tending to be plagued by high blood pressure, diabetes and heart disease.

Clinicians define youngsters as obese if their weight is above the 95th percentile on standard height-and-weight charts. Obesity is surprisingly difficult to treat, since medical scientists don't understand all of the causes. Moreover, therapists have to balance off the benefits of shedding pounds against the possibility of retarding growth.

Against this uncertain backdrop, it *is* known that childhood obesity is commoner these days. The proportion of children who are obese has risen by more than 40 percent just in the last 15 years, according to a study . . . published in the *American Journal of Diseases of Children.* Tests in which the skin is pinched and its thickness measured show that obesity has increased by 54 percent among children age 6 to 11 and by 39 percent among children age 12 to 17, say study authors Steven Gortmaker, a sociologist at the Harvard School of Public Health, and Dr. William Dietz, director of clinical nutrition at the New England Medical Center in Boston.

Fat parents, fat children—usually

Dr. Kenneth Cooper, director of the Aerobics Center in Dallas, sees a future inhabited by unhealthy adults. "I'm afraid that as these kids grow up," he says, "we will see all the gains made against heart disease in the last 20 years wiped out in the next 20 years." Reflecting this concern, the American Heart Association noted last November that 5 percent of youngsters age 5 to 18 have unhealthy cholesterol levels—above 200 milligrams per deciliter of blood. The group urged doctors to check for elevated cholesterol in children who are obese or whose families have a history of heart disease, and suggested a goal of

150 mg. The association recommended low-fat diets and exercise for all children.

In recent years, researchers have dispelled many myths about childhood obesity and pinpointed factors that do play a role. Of these factors, genetics is key. A study of 540 adults adopted as children was published [in 1986] in the *New England Journal of Medicine.* It found that the adoptees' weights as adults strongly correlated with the weights of their biological parents, not their adoptive parents. Heavy parents, in other words, tend to have children who will become heavy. Study author Dr. Albert Stunkard, a psychiatrist at the University of Pennsylvania, says that while genes don't automatically translate into obesity, they do make it easier for the pounds to pile on.

It's likely that an obese adult was an obese child. Overly chubby infants less than 6 months old are more than twice as likely as normal to become obese adults; the risk for obese children age 6 months to 7 years is nearly seven times greater. "The older the obese child, the more probable this child will become an obese adult," says psychologist Leonard Epstein of the University of Pittsburgh School of Medicine.

Some researchers think that overfeeding infants—giving them a bottle too often and starting them on solid foods too early—might lead to obesity later by increasing the number of fat cells in the body. A recent study casts doubt on this theory. Physiologist Douglas Lewis of the Southwest Foundation for Biomedical Research in San Antonio found that female baboons overfed as infants for four months developed larger fat cells, but not more of them. The five overfed baboons were obese at 5 years and had four times more abdominal fat than six normal and four underfed baboons. "I can't say we've proven what happens physiologically as people go through life fat or not fat," Lewis says, "but the fat-cell-number idea is going to have to be looked at more." He advises parents to let infants eat as much as they want, but not to coerce them to eat more. . . .

Sloth and the convenient evils of modern-day life don't help. Dietz speculates that eating fast foods, which tend to be salty and fatty, and watching television can be blamed for much of today's high level of childhood obesity. "American children spend an average of 24 hours a week in front of a TV," he says. "That's time they're not using to play tag, ride a bike or just hang out on the corner—which is probably more energy expensive than sitting in front of the tube."

Accordingly, physical fitness has suffered. A 1986 study of 19,000 youngsters age 6 to 17 for the President's Council on Physical Fitness and Sports turned up these dismal results:

• Teenage girls performed worse than a decade ago in eight of nine fitness-related tasks such as sit-ups, the standing long jump and the 12-minute run.
• Forty percent of boys age 6 to 12 could do no more than one pull-up. Boys from 6 to 10 should be able to do at least two.
• Half of the girls age 6 to 17 and 30 percent of the boys age 6 to 12 could not run a mile in under 10 minutes, far short of the norm of 8 to 9 minutes.

Why care if a child needs 12 or 13 minutes to finish a mile? Because the prepubescent couch potato of today is the fat-farm candidate of tomorrow, says Kate O'Shea, an exercise physiologist with the American Alliance for Health, Physical Education, Recreation and Dance. "There is a definite risk of obesity as children who aren't fit get older, beginning with adolescence," she says. "If there's no change in diet or exercise patterns after the age of 18, as a general rule you'll add 1 pound of body fat and lose the use of about a half-pound of muscle each year as the muscles atrophy. Thirty years after high school, people are 30 pounds heavier because of inactivity."

Specialists in childhood fitness blame the down-trend on a continuing de-emphasis of physical education programs. Fewer than 40 percent of students in grades five through 12 take daily physical-education classes, says O'Shea. While the U.S. has plenty of company else-where—the comparable figure is 46 percent for Canadian students, and France requires physical-education classes only three days a week—all Swedish students, by contrast, take daily physical education through the ninth grade.

Medical specialists can't agree on how or when to treat obese children. Many therapists won't seriously consider treatment until a child has gone far beyond the 95th-percentile bench mark. They worry that dieting can interfere with normal growth and that cyclic patterns of off-and-on dieting may make weight loss more difficult. Kelly Brownell, a psychologist and obesity researcher at the University of Pennsylvania, noted that many of the women he saw in his clinic ate very little but didn't lose weight. He then conducted animal studies in which rats were put on diets and later allowed unrestricted access to food. The second time around, the dieting rats took twice as long to lose weight, and on the unrestricted part of the cycle they regained it three times faster. Brownell suspects that the body perceives dieting as a threat and tries to protect energy stores by slowing its metabolism and releasing hormones and enzymes.

No simple solution

Long-term studies are only beginning to tell therapists what treatments pay off. In one of the first studies, completed [in 1985], Epstein in Pittsburgh used a three-pronged approach: A low-fat, high carbohydrate diet to help take off poundage; an exercise program to work off energy, and behavioral modification to change habits that lead to obesity. For a group of 6-to-12-year-olds 40 percent to 45 percent over their ideal weight, the success rate was highest when the children and their parents—at least one of whom usually was obese as well—worked together. After five years, 33 percent of the children in 25 families treated with this method had kept their weight down to levels considered less than obese. In a second group of 25 families, where the child was working alone, 19 percent succeeded. In the third group of 25 families, in which no specific family member was targeted to lose weight, only 5 percent were not obese. Epstein believes that the success rate could be boosted through improved teaching techniques, parental support, diet and an exercise program.

More research should help chart a path. During the next five years, Brownell will see how dieting affects personality, general health and growth. He'll also study the ways in which cyclic dieting might damage one's ability to lose weight. Work under way elsewhere may soon enable therapists to distinguish between children who will outgrow their obesity and those who need to be treated. But as with adults, there's no shortcut in sight.

—Joseph Carey with Ronald A. Taylor

Source: *US News and World Report* (2 March 1987), pp. 66–67.

HOW MUCH IS TOO MUCH?

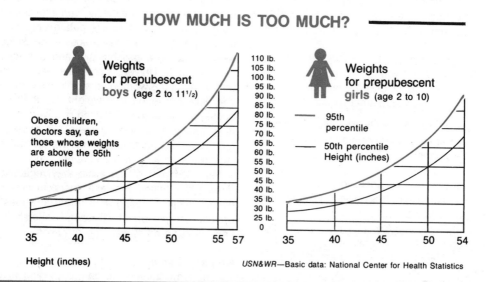

Weights for prepubescent **boys** (age 2 to 11½)

Obese children, doctors say, are those whose weights are above the 95th percentile

Weights for prepubescent **girls** (age 2 to 10)

—— 95th percentile

—— 50th percentile Height (inches)

Height (inches)

USN&WR—Basic data: National Center for Health Statistics

The average weight for both men and women in nearly all age categories has increased since 1960. Women, however, seem to be putting on the pounds faster than men. From 1960 to 1980, the percentage of white women between the ages of 25 and 34 who were obese increased from 13.3 percent to 17.1 percent. During the same time period, the percentage of black women described as obese increased from 28.8 percent to 31 percent. [5] But the problem of obesity is not limited to adults. The proportion of obese children has increased by more than 40 percent in just the last 15 years. [6]

The U.S. Public Health Service recognized the problem of weight control when it established health goals for the 1980s. According to these goals, by 1990 no more than 10 percent of American men and 17 percent of American women should have been more than 20 percent over their desired weight. [7] Unfortunately, this goal was not met. Worse yet, the number of overweight Americans is still growing. The problem is not that people don't want to lose weight, but rather that it is very difficult for most people to make weight loss permanent. Even those who do manage to lose weight tend to gain it back within the first year. Long-term weight reduction and maintenance require major and permanent changes in **life-style**. Many Americans are find it difficult to make and keep such a commitment.

DEFINITIONS

Body weight can be divided into two components: fat weight and lean body weight. **Fat weight** is that portion of body weight attributed to fat or **adipose tissue**. **Lean body weight** is composed of all that remains, the nonfat tissue. This includes bone, muscle, skin, and all internal organs. When discussing **body composition**, keep the following important relationships in mind:

Total Weight = Lean Weight + Fat Weight

Percentage Body Fat = (Fat Weight/Total Weight) × 100

Obesity is an excessive enlargement of the body's total quantity of fat. The actual standards of what constitutes normal levels of fat and what constitutes obesity are somewhat arbitrary. In general, men who have over 20 percent of their total weight composed of fat and women who have over 30 percent of their total weight composed of fat can be considered obese. For example, a 200-pound man, 40 pounds (or 20 percent) of whose body weight was composed of fat, would be considered obese, regardless of his height.

Overweight is a term often used interchangeably with obesity. In fact, the two terms have quite different meanings. Overweight is a statistical concept indicating that an individual weighs more than the norm, or average, for others his or her height and age. This is determined by simply stepping on the scales. The familiar height and weight tables are used to identify individuals who are merely overweight. Since these tables list norms, anyone who is above a given normal range is considered overweight. However, being overweight on the scales does not mean that someone is obese or that his or her body composition is overfat. For example, a weight lifter who develops large muscles will add extra pounds that cause him or her to be overweight according to the height and weight tables. Muscle tissue is more dense and weighs more

(continued on p. 9)

Life-style: A style of living that consistently reflects a particular set of values and attitudes.

Fat weight: The portion of total body weight attributed to fatty tissues.

Adipose tissue: Fat tissue.

Lean body weight: That portion of total body weight that remains after subtracting fat weight, the portion of total body weight attributed to fatty tissues.

Body composition: A breakdown of total body weight into the proportions or amounts attributable to the various components of the body, particularly the 3 major constituents: fat, muscle, and bone.

Obesity: The excessive accumulation of fat in the body to a level that, depending on the age, frame size, and height of the affected person, is considered undesirable.

Overweight: A condition characterized by weight that exceeds what is considered normal and healthy, based on an average taken from people of comparable age, height, frame size, and sex.

Table 1.1 Desirable Body Weight Ranges

MEN					WOMEN				
Height Feet	Inches	Small Frame	Medium Frame	Large Frame	Height Feet	Inches	Small Frame	Medium Frame	Large Frame
5	2	128–134	131–141	138–150	4	10	102–111	109–121	118–131
5	3	130–136	133–143	140–153	4	11	103–113	111–123	120–134
5	4	132–138	135–145	142–156	5	0	104–115	113–126	122–137
5	5	134–140	137–148	144–160	5	1	106–118	115–129	125–140
5	6	136–142	139–151	146–164	5	2	108–121	118–132	128–143
5	7	138–145	142–154	149–168	5	3	111–124	121–135	131–147
5	8	140–148	145–157	152–172	5	4	114–127	124–138	134–151
5	9	142–151	148–160	155–176	5	5	117–130	127–141	137–155
5	10	144–154	151–163	158–180	5	6	120–133	130–144	140–159
5	11	146–157	154–166	161–184	5	7	123–136	133–147	143–163
6	0	149–160	157–170	164–188	5	8	126–139	136–150	146–167
6	1	152–164	160–174	168–192	5	9	129–142	139–153	149–170
6	2	155–168	164–178	172–197	5	10	132–145	142–156	152–173
6	3	158–172	167–182	176–202	5	11	135–148	145–159	155–176
6	4	162–176	171–187	181–207	6	0	138–151	148–162	158–179

The Metropolitan Life Insurance Company tables of desirable weights (copyright 1983, Metropolitan Life Insurance Company) were most recently revised in 1983.

To determine your frame size, extend one arm and bend the forearm upward at a 90 degree angle. Keeping your fingers straight, turn the inside of one wrist toward your body. Then place the thumb and index finger of your other hand on the two prominent bones on either side of your bent elbow. Pull your fingers away while maintaining the space between them. Then measure this space and compare it to the numbers in the table to the right. If your measurement falls within the range listed here, you have a medium frame. If it is smaller, you have a small frame. If it is larger, you have a large frame.

MEN	
Height in 1 inch heels	Elbow breadth
5'2" – 5'3"	$2^{1}/_{2}$" – $2^{7}/_{8}$"
5'4" – 5'7"	$2^{5}/_{8}$" – $2^{7}/_{8}$"
5'8" – 5'11"	$2^{3}/_{4}$" – 3"
6'0" – 6'3"	$2^{3}/_{4}$" – $3^{1}/_{8}$"
6'4"	$2^{7}/_{8}$" – $3^{1}/_{4}$"

WOMEN	
Height in 1 inch heels	Elbow breadth
4'10" – 4'11"	$2^{1}/_{4}$" – $2^{1}/_{2}$"
5'0" – 5'3"	$2^{1}/_{4}$" – $2^{1}/_{2}$"
5'4" – 5'7"	$2^{3}/_{8}$" – $2^{5}/_{8}$"
5'8" – 5'11"	$2^{3}/_{8}$" – $2^{5}/_{8}$"
6'0"	$2^{1}/_{2}$" – $2^{3}/_{4}$"

Note: Weights at ages 25–59 based on lowest mortality. Weight in pounds according to frame (in indoor clothing weighing 5 lbs. for men and 3 lbs. for women; shoes with 1" heels).

Source: Society of Actuaries, and Association of Life Insurance Medical Directors of America, *1979 Build Study*, 1980.

Nearly everyone would like to lose a little weight. Nearly everyone is on a diet, is contemplating beginning a diet or just fell off a diet. Some people even exercise and diet at the same time, a modern form of masochism. To say that Americans are a bit obsessed with weight is to state the obvious.

Perhaps they should be obsessed. By current estimates of obesity experts, 14 million people are 20 percent overweight.

Ideal Weight Is Just an Elbow Away

But how much should someone weigh? It turns out that elbow width is the key. Elbow width determines where you fall in the widely accepted tables of height and weight published by the Metropolitan Life Insurance Company.

If you happen to have big elbows, not fat elbows, but large bony elbows—you can weigh more and feel less guilty about it because you have a large frame and are expected to carry more weight. If the genetic dice throw gave you slender elbows, then you should weigh less because you have a smaller frame. So says the ideal weight table.

But wait. One person's bulk is another's svelte. Ideal weight is a high stakes game in a society in which weight, fitness and diet are tied up in questions of health, long life and self-image. Not surprisingly, the notion of ideal weight generates controversy.

"We don't even like to use the term 'ideal weight' or 'desirable weight' anymore," said Dr. Charles B. Arnold, a medical director at Metropolitan Life. "There are too many interpretations that might be applied."

So the company merely publishes "Height and Weight Tables."

In 1942 and 1959 when Metropolitan published its tables of ideal height and weight based on analysis of millions of life insurance policyholders, the company saw its chart filling a public health education need. It was clear to the actuaries that people who weighed more tended to die sooner. The tables became a standard in the medical profession, giving doctors sound evidence to cite when telling patients that they should drop a few pounds.

Then in 1983, Metropolitan published a new table, again based on statistical analysis of several million policyholders. It listed the weights by age, height and frame size that tended to be associated with living longer. The only problem was that the new weights were higher than those in the older table.

There was an outcry, of course, since Metropolitan seemed to be saying it was suddenly permissible to be a few pounds heavier. "We weren't saying it was alright to be heavier," Dr. Arnold said. "All we were saying was that heavy people seemed to have a lower mortality in 1983 than in 1959 based on study of life insurance policy holders."

Why heavier people might be living longer remains perplexing. Perhaps stopping smoking, controlling diabetes, lowering blood pressure and a gradual shift to less fat in the diet or just better overall medical care are responsible.

But the change in the table highlighted an important truth: There is no definitive way to say exactly what someone should weigh. There are too many variables, ranging from genetic makeup to sociological considerations to a fondness for sandwiches of peanut butter and marshmallow creme.

Still, we all need guidelines with which to whip ourselves onward or provide a cushion of smugness. And nutritionists continue to regard the tables as the best data available.

"I would say the consensus among professionals is that the Metropolitan Life figures are probably as good as any," said Brian Morgan, a Ph.D. nutritionist in the Institute of Human Nutrition at Columbia Presbyterian Medical Center in New York. "Many people in the obesity field would say the numbers probably are too high, but this is a subjective judgment. Nobody really knows what the correct weight for any person is."

The Metropolitan table is based on frame size. Several studies have shown that such things as the size of the elbow, chest, hip, wrist or knee correlate nicely with overall frame size. Metropolitan chose the elbow.

Elbow sizes are best measured with a caliper, which most health clubs or a doctor's office should have. It is also possible to measure your elbow with a ruler. Grasp the two knobby protrusions on either side of the elbow with thumb and forefinger and then have someone measure the distance between the fingers with a ruler.

In each frame category, the height and weight table provides a wide range of acceptable weights.

"In each category I think you should strive to fall in the middle," Dr. Morgan said. "If you're at the upper end of the weight range for your frame size, perhaps you could lose a pound or two. If you're at the bottom, perhaps you should gain a pound or two."

Some sports doctors have an alternative approach to ideal weight based on a formula involving height. A man should take his height in inches, multiply it by four and then subtract 128 to calculate ideal weight. Someone who is 6 feet 2 inches would multiply 74 inches by 4 and subtract 128, coming up with 168 pounds. A woman should multiply height in inches by 3.5 and then subtract 108.

These weights, however, can be low for someone with a large frame, the doctors who use this system say. So they advise adding 10 percent for such people. And who has a large frame? Use a tape measure at the wrist of the dominant hand. For a man, if the wrist circumference is greater than 7 inches, add the 10 percent. For a woman, the circumference would have to be greater than 6^1/$_2$ inches.

Source: William Stockton, *New York Times*, 11 July 1988, sec. 3, p. 11.

than fat, making most muscular people overweight by this definition. Their percentage of body fat may, in fact, be quite low, and the conditioned weight lifter certainly is not obese. As this example illustrates, body composition is the critical factor in determining if a person is obese.

To reinforce the point that fat weight expressed as a percent of body weight determines obesity, we will use the less common but more accurate term, **overfat**, to describe a weight condition that threatens one's health. The term overweight is used only to describe a variation from the statistical norm. Being overweight is not the same as being overfat.

Assessing Body Composition

Assessing body composition is an important first step in a weight-loss program. Without accurate body composition information, a weight-loss goal is at best an educated guess. Once body composition is established, it is possible to determine how much fat must be lost to reach an ideal body weight. Several methods are available to determine what percentage of total body weight is composed of fat.

The most accurate method of determining percentage of body fat is direct chemical analysis. Unfortunately, this is also the least practical because it can be conducted only on cadavers. Direct chemical analysis is of considerable importance, however, because from its use on human cadavers mathematical formulas have been developed that allow us to obtain fairly accurate calculations of body fat by indirect means.

Underwater weighing is usually considered the most accurate of the indirect techniques to determine body fat on live subjects. Over 2 thousand years ago, the Greek mathematician Archimedes determined that a body immersed in fluid experiences a loss of weight equal to the weight of the displaced fluid. Individuals are weighed on a regular scale first and then weighed while underwater in what is commonly called a "dunk tank." Since lean body tissue is more dense than fat, lean individuals will displace more water and will weigh more under water. Using this concept and applying specific mathematical formulas, the percentage of body fat can be determined.

While underwater weighing has been considered the best technique of body composition analysis, there are problems with its use. To calculate body composition with underwater weighing, it must be assumed that lean body tissue and fat tissue each have a constant and unvarying density. For fat, this is largely true. For lean tissue, however, this can be a problem. Black athletes, for

Overfat: Obese, indicating the excessive accumulation of fat in the body.

Underwater weighing: A method of determining amount of body fat using the principle that lean body tissue is denser than fat body tissue. While immersed in water, the lean, denser tissue will displace more water and weigh more than the fat, less dense tissue.

(continued on p. 13)

Here is a physics and fitness lesson: in water, fat floats and muscle sinks. As a result, the vagaries of dieting, ideal weight and the vanities of fitness are turned upside down.

So when someone is perched on a seat suspended from a scale and is holding his breath while submerged in a large tank of warm water in a research laboratory, the readings on the scale are backwards.

Lean vs. Light: Dunking Will Tell

"Ooh, you're nice and heavy," noted Tina Manos, a graduate student at Teachers College of Columbia University, after a research subject being weighed bobs back to the surface, gasping for breath. This is reason for rejoicing, because it means the body is lean and muscular, making it more dense and causing it to weigh more in water.

"Ooh, how light you are," is enough to spark a fit of depression and renewed vows of abstinence at the dinner table. Fat floats.

Manos, who is working on a doctorate in physiology, presides over the hydrodensitometer at the college. It is one of physiology's standard research instruments because it can be used to determine the body's composition: how much of the body is muscle and how much is fat.

Body composition has developed into a specialized field of research recently in terms of fitness, weight control and the study of illnesses related to being overweight. Indeed, researchers are finding that what we weigh is not as critical in health terms as is how much of that weight is lean tissue, or muscle, and how much is fat. Thus, researchers often speak of being overweight in terms more precise than "pounds." They talk about "percent body fat."

So there are people who are both overweight and fat, putting themselves at greater risk for illnesses like heart disease and diabetes. And there are those who are overweight but lean, like weight lifters.

But the ideal in our vain, fitness-crazed world is a third type: normal weight and lean, the leaner the better, according to some.

"The composition of your body rather than your weight alone is emerging as a more important way of looking at how healthy you are," said Bernard Gutin, professor of applied physiology and education at Teachers College. "The proportions of fat versus lean tissue in relation to overall weight is the critical measure."

A study of heart-disease risk factors carried out jointly by Dr. Gutin and colleagues at Mount Sinai School of Medicine and the College of Physicians and Surgeons at Columbia University illustrates body composition's growing importance. The study was published [in 1987] in the Journal of Clinical Investigations.

Carrying too much weight has long been regarded as one of the prime risk factors for developing heart disease. But do people who are overweight because they are muscular rather than fat exhibit heart-disease risk factors different from those of people who are overweight and fat in the traditional way?

The researchers recruited a group of overweight, fat men; a group of normal weight, lean men, and a third group of overweight, lean men.

They classified them in terms of percent of body fat by dunking them in the hydrodensitometer. They then studied other coronary risk measures in each group, such as blood pressure and levels of insulin and cholesterol-related fats in the blood.

They concluded that the overweight but lean men had the same low risk of developing heart disease as the normal weight, lean men. The overweight, fat men were at greater risk.

Similar body-composition studies are under way at a number of laboratories around the country. Many use the hydrodensitometer, and some have begun experimenting with high-tech approaches, such as harnessing some of the radiologist's body-imaging technology to measure bone and tissue density.

But many studies also involve something as simple as using a pair of calipers to measure the thickness of a fold of skin at several points over the body. While not as precise as the hydrodensitometer or the radiological measures, skin-fold thickness measurements produce useful results.

Despite the research, what percentage of body fat is ideal is often debated. Elite athletes, like marathoners, frequently have body fat levels as low as 5 percent. The Mount Sinai and Columbia researchers chose 15 percent body fat and below as their criterion for their lean subjects and 25 percent and above for their fat subjects. Women generally have about 7 to 10 percent more body fat than men, and the percentage of body fat increases with age in both sexes.

When measuring subjects for body fat, Manos begins with calipers and skin-fold thickness tests, taking pinches at the midriff, on the chest just below the shoulder and on the front of a thigh.

Then her subject steps into the large stainless steel tank dressed in a swimsuit, suffering hunger pangs from the overnight fast Manos prefers. (She doesn't want a recent meal to distort the measurements.) Manos teaches how to exhale so as to expel as much air as possible from the lungs, since air is buoyant and can cause someone to float. Then her subject sits on a swing-like perch suspended from a scale. He exhales and then ducks completely under water and stays perfectly still while the scale steadies and she takes a reading.

Manos makes her subjects do this 10 times, looking for several consistent readings.

The moment of truth comes when a printout emerges from a computer and she circles the number labeled "Percent Fat."

Recently, a middle-aged research subject went through the process. Years of being careful about calories and enduring the pain and struggle of countless workouts hung in the balance as Manos scanned the printout.

"Not bad," she murmured, "for your age."

The number she had circled was 15.001.

Source: William Stockton, *New York Times,* 14 November 1988, sec. 3, p. 11.

FIGURE 1.1
Underwater Weighing Technique

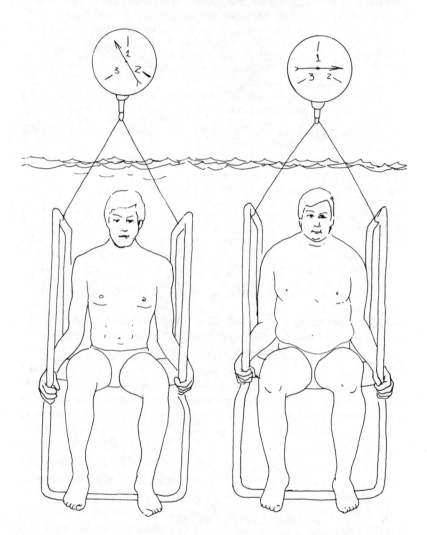

Source: Adapted from J. H. Wilmore and D. L. Costilt, *Training for Sport and Activity* 3d Revised Edition (Dubuque, IA: William C. Brown and Co., 1987), p. 377.

The underwater weighing technique illustrated here is used to determine body composition. Because muscle and body tissue weigh more than fat, two people who are the same height and weight but have different body compositions will have different underwater weights.

example, have been found to have a lean tissue density higher than that of the value typically used in underwater weighing formulas. Also, the composition of lean tissue changes with age because bone mineral and muscle mass have decreased. One would have to adjust the underwater-weighing procedure when assessing these groups to compensate for the differences.

An additional problem with underwater weighing concerns air in the lungs. It is important for subjects being weighed underwater to exhale all the air they possibly can. Since air is lighter (less dense) than water, it tends to make a person weigh less and thus appear more fat. For people who find it difficult to be submerged in water, blowing out all their air and holding still long enough for an accurate reading can be a major problem. An estimate still has to be made of the air left in the lungs, since not all air can be expelled. This calls into question the accuracy of the estimate.

Despite its limitations, underwater weighing still sets the standard to which other techniques are compared. Unfortunately, it is not a practical technique for the average person, since specific equipment and technological know-how are required. The equipment and trained personnel needed to determine body composition through underwater weighing may be available through a local hospital, a health club, or a university health and exercise science program.

Another technique that has gained considerable popularity is **electrical impedance**. A practitioner first places electrodes on one of the subject's toes and an arm. A machine then registers the body's resistance to a low-voltage electrical current that runs between the two electrodes. Since fat tissue and lean tissue conduct electricity differently, a measure of body fat can thus be obtained. This technique is easy to use and creates no discomfort for the subject. However, its accuracy is still in question. Temperature and hydration status can greatly affect results.

Since it is estimated that one-half of the body's total fat content is located immediately beneath the skin, measuring these fat stores is another way of approximating the percentage of body fat. Called **skinfold measurement**, this method involves firmly grasping a fold of skin and **subcutaneous fat** with the thumb and forefinger and pulling it away from the underlying muscular tissue. A special pincer-type caliper exerting a constant amount of tension is used to measure the size of the fold. By obtaining readings at various body sites and comparing these readings to established tables, the percentage of body fat can be calculated. Using skinfolds to determine body fat has distinct

Electrical impedance: A method of determining amount of body fat by measuring the body tissue's resistance to a low-voltage electrical current. This method works on the principle that lean tissue and fat tissue conduct electricity differently.

Skinfold measurement: A method of determining the percentage of body fat by measuring folds of skin from several areas of the body with a specialized caliper.

Subcutaneous fat: A layer of fat found below the skin but over the muscles.

FIGURE 1.2
Skinfold Measuring Technique

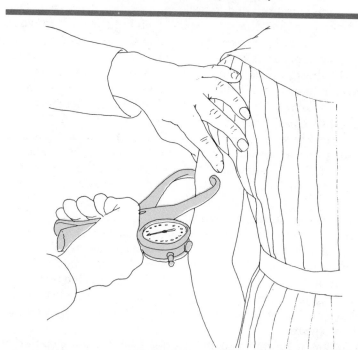

The percent of body fat can be calculated by using a special pincer-like caliper at different locations on the body.

advantages over underwater weighing. The equipment used is uncomplicated and relatively inexpensive, and the technique can be applied almost anywhere. Skinfold measurement also has a drawback, since the person taking the measurements must have considerable expertise in the technique in order to obtain accurate and consistent skinfold values.

A variety of simple formulas is also available to help determine proper weight. These formulas usually are based on height and weight, so they have the same limitations as the traditional height and weight tables. While these formulas can be used to create an awareness of weight problems, they should not be used as the sole means of establishing weight-loss goals.

The best known and most widely used formula to establish obesity is the **Body Mass Index**. This can be calculated by

Body Mass Index: A method of establishing normal weight, grade 1 obesity, or grade 2 obesity through a mathematical formula, using one's weight and height as variables.

FIGURE 1.3
Weight Gain and Body Type

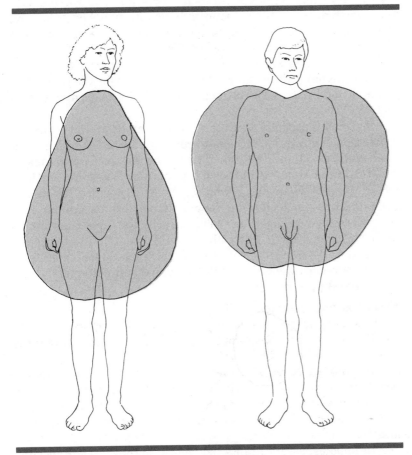

People whose fat is stored in the abdominal cavity area (the "apple shape") have a greater risk of heart disease than those whose fat is stored primarily in the area of the hips and thighs (the "pear shape"). In general, the apple shape is more common among men while women are predominantly pear-shaped.

multiplying one's weight in pounds by 703. Divide the answer by the subject's height in inches. Divide this answer *again* by height in inches. The result is one's body mass index. If the body mass index is 20 to 25, the individual is considered to be of normal weight. Grade I obesity corresponds to a body mass index of 25–29.9; Grade II, of 30–39.9; and Grade III is anything in excess of 40. In the United States, a body mass index of 46–48 is often required by insurance companies for reimbursement of surgical treatment of obesity. [8]

It is possible to determine an approximate ideal weight for men by multiplying height in inches by 4 and subtracting 128. For women, the formula is to multiply height in inches by 3.5 and then subtract 108. Another formula to determine approximate ideal weight instructs men to allow 106 pounds for the first 5 feet of height and add an additional 6 pounds for every inch over 5 feet. For women this formula allows 100 pounds for the first 5 feet of height and adds an additional 5 pounds for each inch over 5 feet.

A final technique that can shed light on obesity and its related health consequences is to compare the measurements of one's waist and hips. The risk of heart disease goes up if a man's waist is larger than his hips or if a woman's waist-to-hips ratio is 0.8 or larger. [9] In other words, people who store fat in the abdominal cavity (called an "apple shape") are at greater risk than persons who store fat primarily in the hips and thighs (called a "pear shape"). Extra abdominal fat contributes to premature artery disease in three ways: It increases blood cholesterol levels, decreases the body's ability to use insulin effectively, and raises blood pressure. [10]

Essential and Storage Fat

Further complicating the issue of proper body composition is the fact that not all body fat is bad. In fact, a certain amount of fat is needed by the body for it to function normally. Body fat can be divided into two types, essential fat and storage fat. **Essential fat** is needed for normal physiological functioning. It is found in the bone marrow, heart, lungs, spleen, kidneys, intestines, muscles, and nervous system. This is not the type of fat one should try to lose.

In females, essential fats include those that are sex specific. Such fat is found, for example, in the mammary glands and pelvic or hip region. Female hormones encourage the stockpiling of this type of fat. In the past, this fat probably served a vital role in reproduction. When women were pregnant or lactating and could not find enough food to eat, this fat was made available to nourish the developing fetus or newborn baby. Today, some women may still need these fat stores if they experience extended periods of morning sickness and nausea. Most women, however, experience less difficult pregnancies and do not need these extra pounds. Nevertheless, these fat stores are built up and maintained, and, because they are metabolically very inactive, they are hard to lose.

Essential fat: One of two major forms of body fat. Essential fat cells maintain normal physiological functioning and are found in bone marrow, the heart, lungs, spleen, kidneys, intestines, muscles, and nervous system.

FIGURE 1.4
Storage Fat Comparisons

Did You Know That . . .

Obstetricians estimate that a pregnant woman's total weight gain should be between 20 and 30 pounds. Gaining less than 20 pounds, or trying to lose weight during pregnancy, can endanger the baby.

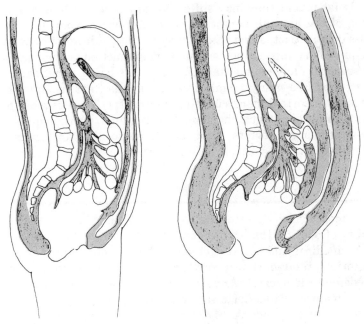

Source: Adapted from *Jane Brody's Nutrition Book* (New York: Bantam Books, 1981) p. 286.

Storage fat (colored areas) is accumulated adipose tissue. This type of fat is usually stored just under the skin surface and around various vital organs. It is valuable as insulation, as protection against injury, and as a reserve of water and fuel in case of emergencies. The overweight person (figure on the right) has an excess of storage fat.

The other major type of body fat, **storage fat**, is accumulated as adipose tissue. This is usually stored just under the skin surface and around various vital organs. Storage fat is valuable as insulation, to protect against injury, and as a reserve of water and fuel in case of an emergency. Unfortunately, the majority of Americans carry much more storage fat than the body needs.

The proportional distribution of storage fat to total body weight in healthy males and females is similar, 12 percent in males and 15 percent in females. However, as a result of sex-specific fat, the total quantity of essential fat in females is 4 times

Storage fat: One of two major types of body fat. Storage fat cells accumulate as adipose tissue.

higher than in males. There seems to be a biologically set minimum level of fat required to maintain good health in both males and females. In males, the lower limit for body fat is about 3 percent of total body weight. For females, this lower limit seems to be around 12 percent of total body weight. One possible sex-specific side effect for females with exceptionally low levels of body fat is that they may suffer **dietary amenorrhea**, a disruption of the normal menstrual cycle that can accompany weight loss or a restricted diet. Exactly what critical level of body fat is required to maintain normal menstrual function is unclear. Some researchers have suggested 17 percent as being a critical level, but there are many female athletes in the 8–13 percent range who have normal menstrual functioning. [11] There is probably a wide range of physical, hormonal, nutritional, psychological, and environmental factors that come into play and must be considered.

OBESITY

The most health-threatening aspect of being overfat is the possibility of obesity. Health dangers linked to this condition include both medical and social problems. Obesity has gained so much notoriety, though, that a counterculture movement has emerged to defend the overfat. Any discussion of obesity has to take this movement and its effects into consideration.

Medical Aspects of Obesity
It is well established that obese individuals—those with an excessive accumulation of fat in the body—are likely to experience more chronic disease and medical complications than their lean counterparts. While the degree to which obesity causes each specific medical problem may not yet be clear, experts agree that obese people face higher health risks than those who are normal weight or less dramatically overweight.

Hypertension, or high blood pressure, is one medical condition related to obesity. If untreated, hypertension can lead to strokes or a variety of other medical complications. While the exact cause of most hypertension is unknown, studies show that obese individuals have a higher risk of suffering this "silent killer." In fact, people diagnosed as hypertensive are often advised to lose weight in order to control the condition.

Obesity has other pronounced effects on the heart and circulatory system. As an individual adds extra pounds of fat, the heart is forced to work harder to pump blood to these additional

Dietary amenorrhea: The absence of menstruation resulting from severe weight loss.

Hypertension: Abnormally high blood pressure.

FIGURE 1.5
Obesity and Health Risks

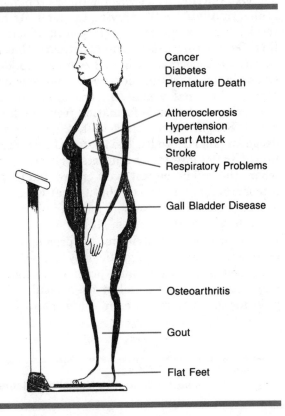

Cancer
Diabetes
Premature Death

Atherosclerosis
Hypertension
Heart Attack
Stroke
Respiratory Problems

Gall Bladder Disease

Osteoarthritis

Gout

Flat Feet

Obese individuals are more likely to experience chronic disease and medical complications than people who are not overweight. Extra weight puts stress on the bones, joints, and organs.

Did You Know That . . .

For those who are truly obese—at least 60 percent heavier than their ideal weight— losing just 10 percent of that weight can help alleviate hypertension, heart disease, and diabetes.

body tissues. In addition, fatty tissue can affect the level of fat in the blood and can lead to **atherosclerosis,** or the buildup of fat deposits in the arteries. Atherosclerosis is related to coronary artery disease and may result in the need for open heart surgery. At the worst, it can even lead to fatal heart attacks.

Current information also suggests that certain types of cancers are related to obesity. In studies conducted by the American Cancer Society, obese men, regardless of smoking habits, were found to have higher rates of colon, rectal, and prostate cancer

Atherosclerosis: A buildup of cholesterol, fat, and cellular debris within the inner layer of the arteries.

than were men of normal weight. Higher mortality rates from cancers of the gallbladder, cervix, uterus, ovary, and breast were found in very obese women.

Osteoarthritis, a type of arthritis common in elderly people, is also associated with carrying extra fat. Arthritis is a disease of the joints. It is characterized by inflammation, pain, and swelling. Osteoarthritis is a form of arthritis that is thought to occur through the normal wear and tear on the joints as people age. Obese individuals put more wear and tear on their joints than people of normal weight. In one study, researchers at Boston University looked at information from the famous Framingham Heart Study, which followed 1,420 persons for more than 3 decades. From this data, the Boston University researchers determined that those study subjects who were obese 36 years ago, when the study began, were more likely to have developed osteoarthritis than those subjects that were not obese. The heaviest 20 percent of the women, for example, were twice as likely to have developed the disease. [12]

Obesity can contribute to problems in pregnancy. Researchers report that significantly overweight women have an increased risk of developing pregnancy-related **diabetes**, which may require a special diet or even insulin treatment to reduce risks for the mother and baby. More than 1 in 4 pregnant women

(continued on p. 22)

Osteoarthritis: A common joint disease among elderly people, resulting from excessive wear on joints, sometimes due to obesity, slight deformity, or misalignment of bones. Common symptoms include pain, swelling, stiffness, joint distortion and enlargement, and weakness of surrounding muscles.

Diabetes: A disorder characterized by abnormally high levels of glucose (sugar) in the blood resulting from the failure of the pancreas to produce a sufficient supply of insulin, the hormone responsible for the conversion of glucose into a form usable by the cells of the body; the major symptoms of diabetes are fatigue, weight loss, excessive urination, and thirst.

Table 1.2 Weight-to-Mortality Relationship

Overweight (percent)	Excess Mortality* (percent)	
	Men	Women
10	13	9
20	25	21
30	42	30

*Compared with mortality of standard risks. Mortality ratio of standard risks equals 100%.
Source: Weight-to-Mortality Relationship, Metropolitan Life Insurance Company, derived from data of the Build and Blood Pressure Study, Society of Actuaries, 1979.

Another table from Metropolitan Life shows that being overweight can be fatal. The figures on the left represent overweight percentage; those on the right show the excess mortality risk such a percentage presents. (All figures are from a 1979 study and are the most recent percentages available.)

FIGURE 1.6
The Three Graces

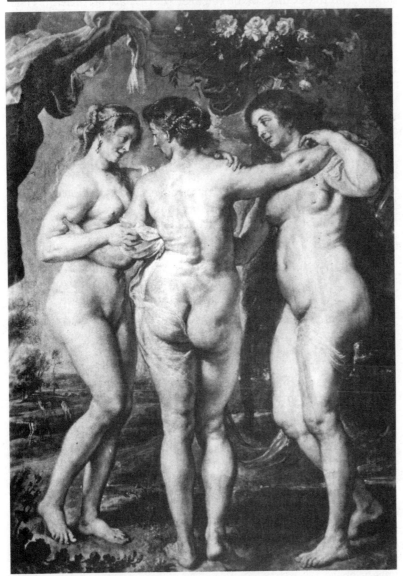

Source: Bettmann Archive.

It has not always been the fashion for women to be thin. In *The Three Graces,*
painted in 1639, Peter Paul Rubens presents his ideal of feminine beauty.

weighing more than 200 pounds have elevated blood pressure. In pregnancy this can lead to a condition called **preeclampsia**, which is characterized by water retention, protein in the urine, and a sharp rise in blood pressure. If preeclampsia is not treated, it can lead to **eclampsia**, or seizures that create significant risks for the mother and baby. Finally, obesity creates problems during labor and delivery. Obese women are more likely to need drugs to augment their labor contractions, and the actual labor time is likely to increase. Obese women are more likely to have large babies. Large babies pose the risk of a more complicated delivery in which the head is delivered but the shoulders get stuck. [13]

A host of other medical problems are also associated with obesity. This list includes gallbladder disease, diabetes mellitus, pulmonary disease, problems with anesthesia during surgery, gout, abnormal **plasma lipid** and **lipoprotein** concentrations, menstrual irregularities, flat feet, intertriginous dermatitis (infections in the skinfolds), organ compression by adipose tissue, and impaired heat tolerance. [14] Finally, many experts believe that obesity can lead to premature mortality.

Social Effects of Obesity

In the past obesity was more socially acceptable than it is today. This can be seen in the paintings of August Renoir and Peter Rubens, which glorified the well-rounded female body. Today, the high-fashion model represents the standard of beauty in the United States. One need not look at many of these young women to realize that fat is no longer considered desirable. Indeed, while this is not the ideal that health professionals would say to emulate, it is far more socially acceptable for women to show no curves at all than to show even the slightest fat deposits. Aspirations for a thin figure, especially when they occur among women, are not without their effect on mental health as well.

Obesity can cause other social problems. Severely overweight people may face job discrimination, both conscious and unconscious. For good reason, certain jobs, in law enforcement, fire fighting, piloting airliners, and the military, for example, have rigid guidelines regarding acceptable body weight. If these guidelines are not met, employment is not possible. While these rules are valid and serve to protect the obese individual and the public, they nevertheless restrict employment opportunities for the severely obese.

Less well known, perhaps, is the fact that, in addition to those professions where weight restrictions are expected, many general employers use weight as a condition of employment

Preeclampsia: A condition of late pregnancy; characterized by high blood pressure, fluid retention, and protein in the urine. If untreated, preeclampsia may lead to eclampsia.

Eclampsia: A condition characterized by a series of seizures during late pregnancy, labor, or the postnatal period; can cause coma or death.

Plasma lipid: Any of the fatty, organic substances carried in the blood plasma, the fluid portion of the blood that remains after the blood cells have been removed.

Lipoprotein: A class of proteins found in the blood that consist of a simple protein combined with a lipid, a class of fatty substances that are insoluble in water, transported throughout the body by the blood, and are one of the body's important sources of food energy.

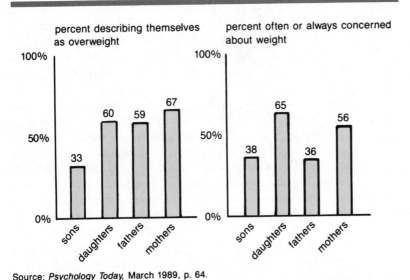

FIGURE 1.7
Weight Anxiety: The Gender Factor

percent describing themselves as overweight

percent often or always concerned about weight

Source: *Psychology Today,* March 1989, p. 64.

Extra pounds worry women more than men, even if both feel overweight.

without ever saying so. While the job description may never mention a weight requirement, it is evident by looking at the work force that obese individuals are not hired. In a study conducted at the University of Pittsburgh, for example, 350 women who each had a master's degree in business administration were surveyed. So few of these women were overweight that the conclusion drawn from the study was that "heavy women tend not to be in management." In the same study, 850 male MBA graduates were surveyed. The results of this survey indicated that those male MBAs who were 20 percent overweight earned roughly $4,000 a year less than their average-weight counterparts. It seems the overweight not only have trouble getting hired but earn less money when employed. [15] Another reason the obese may not be hired, one reinforced by the growing evidence of a health-risk connection to being overfat, is the growing pressure to reduce health-care costs among employees. More than ever, employers are considering the health-related aspects of a potential employee's life-style before making a hiring decision.

Unconscious job discrimination probably accounts for more employment problems for the obese than conscious job discrimination. When two applicants have fairly equal qualifications for a job and one is obese, the employer may opt for the non-obese candidate on the basis of appearance alone without even realizing it. Society has created preconceived notions that obese individuals are slow, lazy, and have little personal control. As corporations strive for efficient, streamlined operations and cultivate the image of the "lean and mean" workforce, the obese simply don't fit in.

Society discriminates against the obese in other ways, too. Seats in theaters, athletic stadiums, airplanes, buses, and even cars are made for people of average weight. To sit in such seats when one is obese is uncomfortable at best and often impossible. Shopping for clothes can be very frustrating for those who carry extra pounds. Store models and fashion displays always use lean individuals that serve to remind the obese that they do not belong. The racks of clothes are often crammed so close together that a lean individual can hardly make it through the aisles, much less someone who is obese. Many times the more attractive styles and colors are not available in large sizes, thereby limiting the selection for large people. When large sizes are available, they are often in a separate section of the store or in a totally separate store, and they often cost more. This further separates and segregates the obese.

Couple these societal problems with the poor body image and poor self-esteem that often accompany obesity, and it is not difficult to understand why obese people are sometimes depressed and unhappy. These negative feelings can be one of the causes of overeating, thus creating a vicious circle where negative feelings lead to overeating, which then leads to obesity, which in turn causes more negative feelings and continued overeating. The psychological effects of obesity are so profound that the Panel on Health Implications of Obesity, formed by the National Institutes of Health, stated, "Obesity creates an enormous psychological burden. In fact, in terms of suffering, this burden may be the greatest adverse effect of obesity." [16]

COUNTERCULTURE MOVEMENT

Recently, we have begun to see a backlash against the cultural norm for thinness. Obese individuals have started to say "It's OK to be fat." Consider television's Nell Carter from *Gimme a Break* and Roseanne Barr from *Roseanne*, professional football's William "Refrigerator" Perry, or the Fat Boys from the world of music. All have used their rotund figures to help propel them to fame. A support organization for the obese has formed. Called the National Association to Aid Fat Americans, its purpose is to inform people that there are also dangers associated with being thin and that fat people can be happy and successful.

The feminist movement has also attacked society's view of obesity and thinness. It has been suggested, for example, that excessive eating, particularly in women, is a direct result of their social position. [17] Women who fit the cultural norm—who are slender and attractive—often feel they cannot be accepted by men as equals. They feel that instead they are being viewed as little more than sex objects. As a result, at a subconscious level they become obese to neutralize their sexual identity. As Susie Orbach says:

> In this way they [women] can hope to be taken seriously in their working lives outside the home. It is unusual for women to be accepted for their competence in this sphere. When they lose weight, that is, begin to look like a perfect female, they find themselves being treated frivolously by their male colleagues. . . . Fat is a symbolic rejection of the limitations of the women's role, an adaptation that many women use in the burdensome attempt to pursue their individual lives within the proscriptions of their social function. [18]

The main point of all these groups and individuals is that obese people should not be concerned with trying to meet society's standards of an ideal weight. Instead, they should accept themselves as they are and get on with more important issues in life. These groups have probably contributed significantly to the mental health of their members and other obese Americans. Unfortunately, the physical problems associated with obesity have not been confronted in any meaningful way by the pro-fat groups. Obesity is a problem that runs across the physical, mental, and social aspects of health, and all three of these aspects need to be addressed in any obesity-related program. It is certainly desirable to remove societal pressure on the obese and to improve their self-concept, but it is equally desirable to reduce body fat to a safe level, one that enhances each individual's health and well-being. W

Did You Know That . . .

Lillian Russell, a popular soprano at the turn of the century, weighed 186 pounds and was considered a great beauty. In contrast, Twiggy, the fashion model superstar of the 1960s, was 5' 7½" and weighed only 91 pounds.

2

Factors Affecting Weight

OBESITY IS A HEALTH PROBLEM charged with conflict. The problem appears simple enough: Obese people eat too much and gain unwanted pounds of fat. The reality is more complex. A myriad of potential causes of obesity have been identified, but they create confusion for anyone interested in really understanding the problem. For example, consider this opening to an article on obesity in the *New England Journal of Medicine* by two doctors:

> There seems to be no end to the contradictory statements made about human obesity. Here are a few. Obesity is the result of a metabolic defect; no, it is no more than the unfettered drive for pleasure derived from eating. Obesity is genetically determined; no, it is the consequence of an abundance of foods and a sedentary life-style. Obesity can be reversed by sensible changes in life-style; no, five-year treatment successes are practically nonexistent. [1]

To examine the confusion that exists, it may be helpful to consider obesity as a group of disorders, not as one disorder affecting millions of victims. It is true that all obese people have one characteristic in common: All of them have an overabundance of fat cells. However, evidence is mounting that the factors causing this excess may differ from person to person. These various factors are the focus of this chapter.

HEREDITY

The effects of heredity on obesity are not clearly understood. While it is true that 75 percent of overweight children have at least one overweight parent, it is not known whether this is because of heredity or environmental conditioning. Supporting the theory of environmental conditioning are studies of identical twins who were separated at birth. These show that the twin raised by overweight parents who pushed food tended to be overweight, while the twin raised by normal-weight parents tended to be of normal weight. [2] These studies, however, cannot be considered conclusive, and evidence is mounting that a genetic factor may in fact exist. One University of Pennsylvania study measured 540 Danish adults who were raised by adoptive parents. The authors of this study found a strong relationship between obesity in adoptees and their natural parents. In contrast, no such relationship was found between adoptees and their adoptive parents. [3] A more recent study examined the effects of overfeeding identical twins. These young adult males were overfed by 100 calories per day, 6 days a week, for a total of 84 days. The average weight gain was 16 pounds. The range was from 8.5 to 26.5 pounds. The similarity of weight gain within each pair of twins was high, while similarities between pairs of twins was low. The authors concluded that the most likely explanation for their findings was that genetic factors were involved. [4] The only logical conclusion to be drawn from the results of the various studies available at this time is that some forms of obesity are probably the result of genetic influences, while other forms are more likely the result of a range of environmental influences.

There is a way to identify those who may be genetically vulnerable to obesity. According to Dr. Albert Stunkard, Director of the Obesity Research Group at the University of Pennsylvania, the best way to make this determination is by looking at a person's family. If both parents are obese, then the subject is vulnerable. If both parents are thin, the subject is less susceptible to the risk of excessive weight gain. Having thin parents, however, does not mean one is free of genetic risk. It is quite possible that thin parents are thin because their efforts to eat well and exercise have overcome a genetic predisposition to obesity. If one parent is lean and the other is fat, there is a clear risk, but how much risk is impossible to say. If obesity runs in a family, however, it does not mean a person should give up and resign himself or herself to being obese. As Stunkard notes:

A great many people whose parents are both overweight have been able to lose weight and stay slim. They may have had to work harder, to eat less and exercise more, but they still did it. [5]

Did You Know That . . .

Babies, adolescents, pregnant women, and tall, thin people have faster metabolism than other people. Men's metabolism is usually higher than that of women because they have more muscle mass.

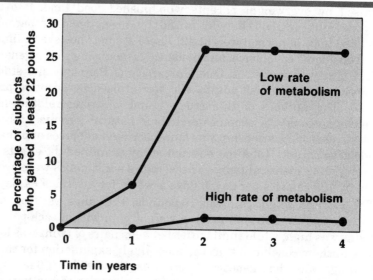

FIGURE 2.1
Metabolism and Obesity

Source: Gina Kolata, "New Obesity Studies Indicate Metabolism is Often to Blame," *New York Times*, 25 Feb. 1988, p. B5, col. 3.

After two years, nearly 30 percent of the subjects [in a *New England Journal of Medicine* study] who had low rates of metabolism when fasting, had gained at least 22 pounds. In contrast, fewer than 5 percent of the subjects with high metabolic rates had gained that much weight. Metabolism is the process by which the body transforms food into energy. With slower metabolism, less food is burned as energy and more becomes body fat.

METABOLISM

Metabolism: The physical and chemical process whereby the body transforms food into energy by breaking large molecules into smaller molecules.

For years obese people have expressed frustration at their inability to lose weight and at their tendency to regain weight quickly. While many of these obese people questioned whether their weight problems might be related to **metabolism**, the amount of energy required to perform normal daily functions, weight-control experts tended to dismiss such physiological causes of obesity. They emphasized instead the psychological causes that led to becoming overfat and the effect of over-consumption of food. The validity of studies that indicated obese people ate no more than their lean counterparts was often questioned. It was even sug-

(continued on p. 30)

For those who have struggled to lose weight or keep it off, research into the origins of obesity has begun to offer an absolution of sorts. [In 1988] two studies published in the *New England Journal of Medicine* showed that some fat people, rather than being slothful or gluttonous, have an inborn predisposition to gain weight. Reason: instead of burning off excess calories as others do, obese bodies are pro-

Is Losing Weight a Losing Battle?

grammed to convert them into fat. Thus, while fat people may eat the same amount of food as thinner people do, they gain more weight. Moreover, their tendency to get fat is probably hereditary.

Researchers have long suspected that a metabolic problem underlies obesity, but until now the evidence has been ambiguous. The studies are the first to have focused on people before they became fat and monitored them as they gained weight. The major finding: certain measurements of metabolism, such as the rate at which the body consumes oxygen and produces carbon dioxide, can be used to predict who is likely to become obese. Says Dr. George Bray, an obesity specialist at the University of Southern California: "It's the predictive nature of this work that is so important."

A team from the National Institutes of Health found a link between low metabolism rates and excessive weight gain over a period of several years. Their subjects were 171 Pima Indians in Arizona, a tribe in which two-thirds of the women and half the men are obese. Though there were variations among individuals, researchers generally found that the slower the metabolism, the greater the weight gain. Yet after a gain of between 20 lbs. and 45 lbs., metabolism rates changed, rising to a new level.

What does it mean? Some people, it appears, are programmed by their genes to store fat instead of burn it. Scientists speculate that this ability may be a vestige of early human history, when those who could live off their fat reserves were more likely to survive droughts and famines. The bodies of such individuals actively resist every effort to slim down. Below a certain weight, their metabolism slows in order to allow fat to accumulate, but their appetites remain undiminished. Once body weight rises to a certain point, the metabolism seems to speed up, so that they maintain that weight without gaining any more. But, researchers note, a sluggish metabolism does not explain all obesity. Overeating and lack of exercise also seem to play a role in getting fat.

The second study supported the idea that people inherit physiological traits that predispose them to obesity. A group led by Physiologist Susan B. Roberts of Tufts University studied 18 infants during their first year of life: six of their mothers were thin; twelve were overweight. Roberts and her colleagues measured how many calories the babies took in and how many they burned off. By three months of age, six of the babies with overweight mothers were generating 21% less energy than the rest. At one year, the six had become overweight, although they ate no more than the thinner babies.

Researchers, however, were unable to pin down the reason that some infants seemed to expend less energy than others. Their educated guess: babies who gained too much weight were less active than those who didn't. The obvious conclusion: even for infants, exercise is probably the best medicine for obesity. The prescription for adults is the same. The new findings may lift some of the blame for being fat from the obese, but not the responsibility. In certain people, the tendency to put on fat never wanes, and only a life of dieting and exercise can thwart it.

—*Denise Grady. Reported by Suzanne Wymelenberg*

Source: *Time* (7 March 1988), p. 59.

gested that obese people, either consciously or unconsciously, underreported their food intake. With the development of better techniques to study metabolism, however, new evidence is being found to support the role of abnormal metabolism as a cause of some cases of obesity.

One such study recently examined a population of southwestern American Indians known as the Pima. As a group, these people have a higher than normal rate of obesity; two-thirds of the women and half of the men are obese. Recent findings have indicated that, among tribe members, the slower the metabolism, the greater the weight gain. Why should this group of persons exhibit such high rates of obesity? While no one knows for sure, it has been suggested that obesity may have been an important factor in the survival of these people. The sad history of these Native Americans is one of starvation. Perhaps those persons who had slower metabolisms and were able to store significant amounts of body fat were better able to survive the lean times. Through the years, the characteristic of slow metabolism has been passed from generation to generation, creating a group of people today that have inherited a propensity to become obese. [6]

YO-YO EFFECT

In addition to inheriting low metabolism, some people may actually lower their metabolism through dieting. It is common among obese men and women to hear tales of struggling to lose weight and then of gaining the lost pounds back shortly after reaching a more desirable weight. The next time they try to lose weight, it seems even harder to take off and even easier to put back on. This up-and-down body weight phenomenon, not limited to the overfat, has been termed the **yo-yo effect**. It is now believed that the yo-yo type of dieting can actually lower the

---

Losing weight seems to get harder all the time. Maybe that's because the more often you start a new diet, the more your body resists shedding excess pounds. At least that is the belief of a number of leading obesity researchers, including Kelly Brownell, PhD, a professor of psychiatry at the University of Pennsylvania School of Medicine, who is gathering evidence of the "yo-yo" effect of dieting on both animals and human beings.

The Off-Again, On-Again Effect of Repeated Dieting

In a study with laboratory rats, for example, Dr. Brownell observed that after the animals regained weight they had lost when they were placed on a reducing regimen, it took them more than twice as long to lose it the second time around, even though the number of calories they were fed on the weight-loss diet had not been changed. And it took less than one-third the time to gain it back! Specifically, the animals lost their excess weight in 21 days on the first try and regained it in 45 days. But it took 46 days to shed the extra weight when the weight-loss diet was repeated and only 14 days to put it back on again. The difference is thought to be due to a slowdown in the metabolic rate. The body may respond to repeated efforts at weight loss by automatically lowering its metabolic rate to defend against what it interprets as too much starvation. (To conserve energy under the stress of true starvation, the body does actually lower its metabolic rate and thereby expends fewer calories.) In preliminary research on high-school and college wrestlers, Dr. Brownell has found that those who lose and gain pounds frequently to "weigh in" to a desired weight category have significantly lower metabolic rates than the wrestlers whose weights fluctuate little.

Does all this mean that if you have gained back any weight you once lost you should give up the idea of trying to lose it again? Of course not. But it does mean that once you have successfully gone through the effort of losing excess pounds, you should try to continue to develop eating habits that will enable you to keep them off. Slimming down is difficult enough the first time around. No one needs to put himself or herself through an even more difficult second trial.

Source: *Tufts University Diet & Nutrition Letter,* Vol. 5, No. 9, November 1987, p. 1.

Yo-yo effect: Rapid up-down-up weight fluctuations, a phenomenon common among dieters.

Did You Know That . . .

Scientists say the brain chemical serotonin influences appetite. Eating carbohydrates produces serotonin, which makes us feel satisfied. Chronic overeaters may have too little of this chemical.

FIGURE 2.2
The Yo-Yo Effect

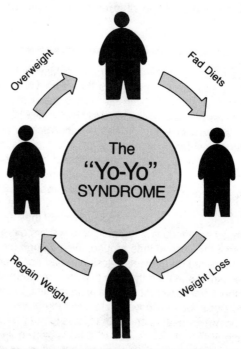

Source: Ferguson, *Diet Center Program* (Little, Brown & Co., 1983) p. 24.

The "Yo-Yo" syndrome of alternately losing and regaining weight is often a result of fad dieting. It is now believed that yo-yo–type dieting can actually lower the metabolic rate of the dieter over time, making it increasingly difficult to lose weight and keep it off.

Metabolic rate: A term used to describe the body's rate of metabolism, a general term for all of the chemical and physical processes that take place continuously within the living body.

metabolic rate of a dieter over time, making it increasingly more difficult to lose weight and keep it off.

Evidence of this effect was seen initially in laboratory rats. The rats were placed on a low calorie diet and forced to lose weight. They were then allowed to eat all they wanted until they had regained the weight they had originally lost. The second time they were placed on a diet, calories had to be further restricted to achieve the same weight loss as the first time. Regaining their weight was easier the second time. It has been theorized that the animals' bodies were trying to protect themselves from starvation by burning calories more slowly.

Evidence of this same phenomenon in humans exists too. Consider a study done on high-school wrestlers. Wrestlers were chosen because it is common practice for them to lose large amounts of weight in a short period of time to make a desired weight class. The metabolic rates of 27 high-school wrestlers were studied during a summer wrestling camp. None of the boys were currently dieting to reduce weight, but half of the boys had lost and regained at least 10 pounds on at least 10 occasions during the regular winter wrestling season. The remaining boys kept their weight steady during the season. Although no differences in percentages of body fat were observed between the dieters and nondieters, the dieters had a 14 percent lower metabolic rate in the off-season. It was hypothesized that this lower metabolic rate was because of the on-and-off dieting of wrestlers in the frequent weight-loss group. [7]

The time period required to lower metabolism through dieting is fairly short. An average-size woman who has never dieted can lower her metabolism by 15 percent in just 3 weeks by eating fewer than 800 calories a day. If she has dieted often in the past, she may be able to obtain the same 15 percent reduction in metabolism in as little as one week. Evidence from anorexic women, who lack or lose their appetite for food, indicates that metabolic rates can be reduced as much as 30 to 40 percent over time with continued starvation. It takes a healthy 100-pound woman 1,000 calories a day to maintain her weight. An anorexic 100-pound woman can maintain her weight on as few as 600 calories a day. [8]

SETPOINT THEORY

Another metabolism factor that may affect long-term weight loss is the **setpoint theory**. Proponents of a setpoint theory believe that the body has an internal control mechanism, probably somewhere in the brain's **hypothalamus**, that predetermines a particular level of body fat for each person. This predetermined body-fat level would probably equal the percentage of body fat maintained if a person were not restricting caloric intake. From a practical point of view, this would mean that when people manage to reduce their body-fat level below the predetermined setpoint, their bodies will make internal adjustments to resist the change and to conserve body fat. In other words, their metabolism will probably be reduced.

Setpoint theory: The hypothesis that the body has an internal control mechanism, centered in the brain, which strives to maintain the individual's predetermined body fat level.

Hypothalamus: A region of the brain located immediately below the thalamus and behind the eyes which regulates the portion of the nervous system that controls the internal organs of the body; the hypothalamus plays a major role in the regulation of body temperature, the so-called "fight or flight" response, and a broad range of other important functions.

Setpoint theorists believe that the best and safest way to affect the setpoint and lower it toward a more desirable level is through regular and sustained vigorous exercise. The main difference between fat people and lean people is usually not how much they eat, but how much they exercise. When obese people exercise regularly, their food intake usually declines despite the increase in caloric output. The result is a decrease of body fat. Eventually, if exercise is maintained, caloric intake balances with daily energy requirements. Body weight stabilizes, and a new, lower setpoint is established. [9]

ADIPSIN ENZYME

Adipsin: An enzyme produced by fat cells and circulated by the blood that is thought to influence the body's appetite control and energy expenditure.

Recent animal experiments have indicated the presence of an enzyme, **adipsin**, that is produced by fat and circulated in the blood. Adipsin affects appetite control and/or energy expenditure and is found in abnormally low levels in certain types of obesity. [10]

The discovery of adipsin plays a very important role in the overall battle against obesity. It marks the first time obesity has been related to abnormal genetic functioning. Scientists have discovered from laboratory research that mice that are genetically predisposed to obesity appear to have low levels of adipsin. Normal mice that have simply been overfed to produce obesity show no change in adipsin levels. [11] If the same holds true in humans, doctors might be able to distinguish obesity that arises from a genetic shortage of adipsin from obesity that results from overeating and underexercising simply by measuring the amount of adipsin present. It has also been suggested that in the future it may be feasible to treat affected obese people with doses of adipsin to enhance normal metabolism. At this point, however, diagnosing and treating obesity with adipsin is pure speculation. Much more research needs to be done before any such treatments could begin. [12]

Fat cell theory: A hypothesis suggesting that the body increases the quantity of fat tissue in two ways: hypertrophy and/or hyperplasia.

FAT CELL THEORY

Hypertrophy: One of two ways fat cell theory suggests that the body increases its fat tissue, by enlarging fat cells that already exist in the body.

In addition to the total percentage of body fat, the actual number and size of fat cells in the body may be an important factor in obesity. This possibility has given rise to a new theory, **fat cell theory**, which suggests that the body increases the quantity of fat tissue in two distinct ways. The first, called **hypertrophy**, is by enlarging existing fat cells. The second, labeled **hyperplasia**,

Hyperplasia: One of two ways fat cell theory suggests that the body increases its fat tissue, by increasing the number of fat cells in the body.

is by increasing the total number of fat cells. Obese people tend to have both more and larger fat cells than non-obese people.

Once a person has an overabundance of fat cells, that number remains fairly constant. When the obese person loses weight, the body fat he or she loses comes from reducing the content of existing fat cells, not from reducing the number of fat cells. This

(continued on p. 37)

Fat-Cell Protein Is Implicated in Obesity

In a major advance in the study of obesity, researchers have discovered that abnormally low levels of a protein produced by fat cells may be linked to the propensity to gain weight.

Unlike other substances made by fat cells, the protein, adipsin, is secreted directly into the blood stream. From the blood, it can get to the brain, possibly affecting appetite or metabolism. It could also directly affect the metabolism of cells elsewhere in the body.

But the most intriguing finding is that animals that are obese for genetic or metabolic reasons make much less adipsin than those of normal weight or those that are obese only because they have purposely been fed too much rich food. Mice with a genetic tendency to obesity, either from low metabolism or from inherited eating patterns, exhibit low adipsin levels, researchers have found.

"It's very exciting," said Dr. Jules Hirsch, a researcher at Rockefeller University in New York. "We're always looking for an elusive signal from the fat cells that relates to eating behavior."

Researchers speculate that some forms of obesity—20 percent or more above ideal body weight—may be tied to a lack of adipsin.

The link between levels of the protein and obesity has been established only in animals so far, but researchers have also found adipsin in humans and are investigating a possible link.

In the past few years researchers have demonstrated that some people inherit a strong tendency to become obese. They believe the inability to make enough adipsin may be a crucial component in obesity that is inherited.

Most recently, researchers have found that the protein closely resembles a protein of the immune system. They believe this finding may help understand how the fat cell protein works.

Bruce M. Spiegelman of the Dana Farber Cancer Center in Boston and his colleagues found that the fat cell protein is nearly identical to a protein of the immune system, known as complement D, that had not been suspected of playing any role other than defending the body against infections. Dr. Spiegelman reported this discovery at a New York meeting on obesity. Dr. Spiegelman and his colleague, Dr. Jeffrey S. Flier of Beth Israel Hospital in Boston, discovered the protein several years ago. The fat cell protein is called adipsin because it is made by adipocytes, or fat cells.

One possibility the scientists are investigating is that adipsin signals the brain to control eating by diminishing appetite and that it may be possible to treat obesity by giving people adipsin. But Dr. Spiegelman said, "This is rank speculation."

To test this theory and others, Dr. Spiegelman and his colleagues are now giving fat animals adipsin to see if they lose weight.

Although the connection between adipsin and complement D was a surprise, researchers noted that other immune system proteins found in recent years also act on the brain.

Until now, the only known relationship between body fat and the immune system was an immune system protein discovered several years ago by Anthony Cerami of Rockefeller University. The protein, which he called cachexin, causes fat loss and wasting. Other researchers then discovered that cachexin is tumor necrosis factor, a natural cancer-fighting hormone made by white blood cells.

The new finding is also making experts look

again at complement D, one of 30 proteins known collectively as the complement system, a part of the immune system. Complement D "punches holes in bacteria," Dr. Spiegelman said.

Nobody has ever associated any of the complement proteins with obesity, said Dr. John E. Volanakis, a complement expert at the University of Alabama who collaborated with Dr. Spiegelman and with Barry S. Rosen of Dana Farber Cancer Center.

Dr. Volanakis said the first clue that adipsin might resemble complement D came when Dr. Spiegelman and his colleagues found that about 60 percent of the amino acids that make up adipsin are identical to the amino acids that make up complement D. In laboratory experiments he found that adipsin acted exactly like complement D in terms of function.

Dr. Spiegelman and Dr. Flier discovered adipsin while looking for molecular signals that turn some mouse skin cells into fat cells, a phenomenon occurring only in the laboratory.

They found a gene that directs the cells to make adipsin, and then discovered adipsin itself. Although adipsin did not regulate the conversion of the skin cells to fat cells—it is made after the cells have already started to turn into fat cells—it turned out to be intriguing for other reasons.

"We learned that adipsin is secreted by fat cells and pumped into the bloodstream," Dr. Spiegelman said. "That was unusual. It is the only protein made by fat cells that freely circulates and it could theoretically connect with the brain and appetite and metabolism."

About [two years] ago, Dr. Spiegelman and Dr. Flier looked at the production of adipsin in obese and normal rats and mice and discovered strong hints that adipsin might play a crucial role in obesity. In these studies, they included animals that were obese for genetic reasons, normal animals that the researchers made obese chemically by destroying a part of the hypothalamus that includes an appetite control center, and normal animals that the researchers made obese by overfeeding.

Normal animals and animals that were obese because they ate too much made 100 to 200 times as much adipsin as the animals that were genetically obese or obese because their hypothalamus had been partially destroyed. Some animals with low adipsin levels became obese from eating too much and others became obese from having slow metabolisms.

Dr. Hirsch said that because the animals with low adipsin constituted a heterogeneous group, including those with several types of genetic obesity as well as the group whose obesity arose from brain lesions, the low levels of the protein must tie in with obesity itself, not the specific kind of obesity.

"On the one hand, this could distinguish obese animals from lean, and on the other hand it could distinguish certain kinds of obesity from each other," Dr. Spiegelman said.

"Adipsin seemed to distinguish those who were obese for dietary reasons from those who were obese because of their metabolisms," he added. "What this is telling you is that there is some pathway in obesity that leads directly to the fat cells themselves."

To learn whether similar findings hold true in humans, Tyler White and his colleagues at Metabolic Biosystems Inc., a subsidiary of California Biotechnology Inc. in Mountain View, Calif., looked for adipsin in people. They found it.

Now, said Karen Talmadge, director of diabetes and obesity research at the company, the group is starting to examine adipsin levels in people of normal weight, those who are obese and from obese families, and those who became obese later in life and have no family history of obesity.

Most obesity researchers think there are many kinds of human obesity, as there are kinds of animal obesity, and that some obese people inherit a strong predisposition to become fat.

"Clearly, we would love it if adipsin turned out to be important in obesity," Dr. Talmadge said. "We hope adipsin will tell us about obesity and we would love to be able to treat obesity by giving people adipsin."

Source: Gina Kolata, *New York Times*, 3 January 1989, sec. 3, pp. 1, 9.

FIGURE 2.3
Fat Cells and Body Weight

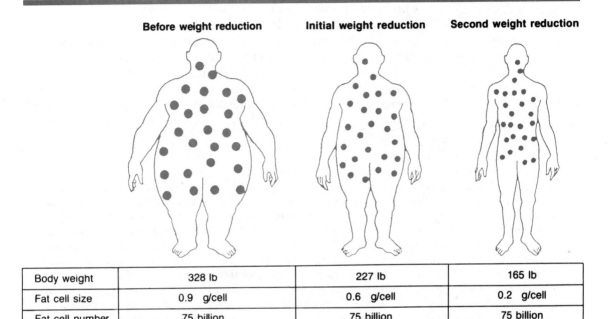

	Before weight reduction	Initial weight reduction	Second weight reduction
Body weight	328 lb	227 lb	165 lb
Fat cell size	0.9 g/cell	0.6 g/cell	0.2 g/cell
Fat cell number	75 billion	75 billion	75 billion

Source: G. H. Stollerman, ed., *Advances in Internal Medicine,* Vol. 17 (Chicago: Year Book Medical Publishers, 1971).

When obese people lose weight, their fat cells shrink in size but not in number. Therefore, a 165-pound man can have the same number of fat cells as a 328-pound man.

larger number of now relatively empty fat cells in the formerly obese individual may have severe implications for maintaining the new weight. It has been suggested that these small fat cells are like empty containers waiting to be filled up. They cause the appetite-control center in the brain to crave more food to fill the starving fat cells. If this is true, the fat cell theory may also be related to the "yo-yo" cycle of weight loss which, as we have noted, is not limited to the overfat. [13]

LACK OF EXERCISE

Lack of regular exercise, or sustained inactivity, appears to be one of the more significant factors related to obesity. No one can definitely determine whether a lack of activity causes obesity or obesity causes a lack of activity, and such a distinction is probably unnecessary. What is true, however, is that those who participate in a regular exercise program are less likely to experience problems related to obesity. In fact, exercise may be the most important factor in the prevention of obesity.

The relationship between activity and obesity appears early in life. Studies have revealed that as early as 3 months after birth, infants that became overweight were less active than their non-overweight counterparts. Total energy expenditure was 20.7 percent less in the infants that became overweight. [14] The same is apparently true of adolescents. Noted nutritionist Jean Mayer has reported:

> Inactivity is indeed the major factor in perpetuating obesity in many, if not most, overweight youngsters. Examination of the dietary intake of equal groups of overweight and normal weight girls, matched for age and height, showed that the obese students fell into two groups. One group, and by far the larger, contained girls who ate no more than the normal weight girls but who exercised considerably less. All the "sitting" activities were emphasized at the expense of the walking and active sports. Television watching consumed four times as many hours in this group as it did in the normal weight group. The second group (the existence of which emphasized the fact that there is more than one cause of obesity) ate more than the normal and exercised normally. These were of the red-cheeked, cheerful type and while "overweight," they appeared less "overfat" than the inactive group. Other studies indicate that the same situation prevails with boys as well. [15]

AGE AND OBESITY

Age is a factor indirectly related to obesity. It has been observed that as Americans age, their amount of body fat tends to increase. Two age-related factors may help to explain this tendency. Typically, as people get older, the amount of physical activity they engage in decreases. Unless accompanied by a proportional decrease in calories, weight gain will occur. Usually this takes place over time, so that one will gain a few extra pounds each year and not be aware that a decrease in physical activity is the cause. Occasionally, however, when an athlete suddenly stops training

FIGURE 2.4
Age and Increasing Weight

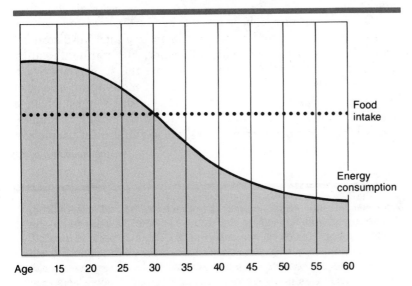

Food intake

Energy consumption

Age   15   20   25   30   35   40   45   50   55   60

Source: Adapted from *American Medical Association Family Medical Guide* (New York: Random House, 1987).

As you grow older, your body seems to need less energy, partly because you become less active, and partly for other reasons not yet clear. But many people do not reduce their food intake to correspond with their decreasing energy requirements. The end result is a calorie surplus that shows up as increasing deposits of fat as you age.

or someone with a physically active job is transferred to a desk job, the result is more immediate and more obvious.

Along with a reduction of exercise, metabolism declines with age. Once again, extra pounds will be added unless caloric intake is proportionally reduced. At age 30, a person's basic caloric need is 10 percent less than that of a 15-year-old. From age 30 on, the average person will need 7 percent less food for each decade of life. [16]

Until recently, weight-loss experts pretty much dismissed the possibility that obesity could be a physiological disorder. Even when such causes were recognized, their importance was downplayed by estimates that as few as 2 to 5 percent of obese persons had physiological problems that explained their condition. Today, however, it seems the evidence is growing to support the existence of a variety of physiological factors related to obesity.

Although experts do not know how many people suffer from genetically and/or metabolically induced obesity, it is probably more than the previously estimated 2 to 5 percent of the population.

On the other hand, obese persons have often been too quick to blame their weight problems on metabolic or glandular disorders. Typically, obese people go on diet after diet, with minimal results. Metabolism, glands, and heredity become the scapegoats to explain fad diets that do not work, a lack of motivation, a lack of exercise, or a host of other problems that limit success. Even if one has a predisposition to obesity caused by heredity or metabolic problems, experts know enough to say that most people can

(continued on p. 42)

D. wants to lose weight, immediately. Since he finds exercise difficult, boring and time-consuming, he decides to take the easy route—he stops eating. He enjoys immediate success: pounds begin to drop off, almost one a day. Unfortunately, D. is not really up to celebrating. He feels tired and depressed and is constipated and frequently cold. Soon, his skin and hair become dry, and he has trouble sleeping at night. Worst of all, he stops losing weight, even though he has continued to eat less than one meal a day. Frustrated and discouraged, D. goes back to his original eating habits. Two weeks later, D. has not only gained back all the weight he lost, but he has even added a few more pounds. Now D. is really depressed.

The Paradox of Dieting

If this fictitious scenario sounds too familiar, you—along with an estimated 90 percent of all crash dieters—have fallen victim to winning the battle of quick weight loss while losing the war of permanent weight reduction: most dieters regain their lost weight within two years.

Why does this happen? Why do you suddenly stop losing weight, and then, when you start eating "normally" again, gain back more than you lost? According to Dr. Wayne Callaway, an obesity specialist at the Mayo Clinic, a few related theories help to explain what's going on.

One theory has to do with your body weight's own natural "set point"—the point at which your weight remains if you make no attempt to lose weight. When you try to maintain a weight below your set point, your body adaptively responds by preparing for semi-starvation: insulin levels drop, and the functioning of the thyroid and catecholamine hormones are altered, causing reductions in pulse rate, respiratory rate, blood pressure, oxygen consumption and carbon dioxide production. Cold intolerance, dry skin and hair, and constipation also result.

the ill effects of fad diets.

According to this theory, the discomfort associated with these symptoms—plus continual hunger—drive the dieter to eat more until the weight is regained.

Meanwhile, according to another theory, when you diet, your metabolic rate—the rate at which you burn calories—slows significantly, which causes the few calories you consume to last longer. But, you might ask, if the body is burning less fat, how is it that some people can lose as much as 20 pounds in the first two weeks of a crash diet? Because, says Callaway, between half and three-quarters of this weight loss is due to "starvation diuresis," or loss of body water. (The more obese you are, the more water you retain.) Your body weight levels off somewhat after about two weeks of dropping water weight; with a slow metabolic rate, actual fat loss amounts to only about a pound or two a week. This also explains why, when you start eating again, you regain all the weight you lost, and just as quickly: it's almost all water.

Why do you frequently gain back *more* than you lose? Again, because you're burning calories at a slower rate than before you started dieting; the same number of calories translates into more fat on your body. Within a month, however, your metabolic rate will return to what it was previously.

Now, before you start justifying last night's double dessert with a quick "diets don't work anyway," remember: we have just explained what occurs when you undertake a crash diet—under 800 calories a day. What works better than any diet, according to Callaway, is a change in eating habits. Callaway suggests eating three balanced meals a day; skipping a meal lowers your metabolic rate, while eating actually raises it. For moderately overweight women, Callaway recommends eating about 500 calories a day less than the total amount of calories you burn during the day, at rest and during physical activity; for more severely overweight women and for overweight men, between 500 and 1000 calories less. This will prevent a dramatic decline in metabolic rate and water weight and diminish alterations of other bodily functions.

To speed up the weight-loss process, regular exercise must be added to the regimen. Since exercise increases your metabolic rate, you burn more calories not only while you exercise, but for several hours after exercising. Added to this, vigorous exercise can decrease your appetite immediately afterwards. How much can you expect to lose on this combined food reduction and exercise program? About a pound a week, the doctor says. But, he warns, don't weigh yourself every day. Daily weight changes are meaningless in terms of actual fat loss; they almost entirely reflect changes in fluid balance. Even weekly weight changes can be misleading. For a more accurate assessment, check the scale every six weeks.

Source: *Consumers' Research,* April 1985, p. 14.

overcome the problem with hard work, proper diet, and plenty of exercise.

"The Diet Mentality" is another problem to consider when discussing long-term weight loss. It stems from the mind-set people usually have when they begin a diet. Most people who "go on a diet" desire quick results and anticipate the day when their goal is finally obtained so they can go back to eating a "normal" diet. This thinking sets up the dieter for failure because as soon as he or she returns to a "normal" diet, he or she is going to gain the weight right back. A better way to think of weight loss is to see it as a life-style change: to undertake a new way of approaching food, eating, and exercise, one that must be maintained over a lifetime. This does not mean that there will not be occasions to eat a double-layer chocolate cake or a banana split. It is unrealistic to think that such treats can never be tasted again. It does mean that this cannot be done on a regular basis. It is of utmost importance that healthy food choices, low in fats and sugars and high in fiber, be the mainstays of one's diet. "Eat to live" is the appropriate motto, not "live to eat." W

3

Weight Control and Exercise

I N ITS SIMPLEST FORM, weight control is a matter of balancing energy input with energy output. In other words, one can maintain one's present weight if the amount of **calories**, or fuel, taken in equals the amount of calories (fuel) used by the body for normal physiological functioning plus exercise, if any. This is a state known as **caloric balance**. However, if caloric input exceeds caloric output, weight will be gained at the rate of approximately one pound for each 3,500 excess calories. Conversely, if output is greater than input, weight will be lost at the rate of one pound for each excess 3,500 calories expended. This holds true regardless of metabolic or hereditary tendencies to maintain or gain body fat. The obvious problem, therefore, is how to obtain the desired state of energy or caloric balance—or imbalance, as the case may be?

Gaining excess fat is a matter of taking in more calories than the number used over an extended period of time. The difference between caloric input and output does not have to be great for gradual weight gain to occur. If a person were to consume 1 extra tablespoon of butter or margarine (100 calories) each day for 1 year, his or her theoretical weight gain would exceed 10 pounds. As long as input exceeds output, weight gain will continue. Eventually, however, the energy requirements of the body will increase because the body is carrying several extra pounds of fat. Energy balance will again be achieved but at a higher level than before.

Take, for example, the hypothetical and oversimplified situation of Gary, who currently looks slim and trim and has a low percentage of body fat. He takes in 2,500 calories and uses 2,500 calories each day, so he is in a state of caloric balance. He is

Calorie: The most widely used measure of the energy content of foods, the term calorie is actually an abbreviated version of the more technically correct term, kilocalorie or kcal, defined as the amount of heat necessary to raise the temperature of one *kilogram* of water one degree Celsius at normal atmospheric pressure; sometimes confused with the "small calorie" used in physics and chemistry; the latter equals the amount of heat necessary to raise the temperature of one *gram* of water by one degree Celsius at normal atmospheric pressure.

Caloric balance: When one's caloric intake is equal to the number of calories one expends in maintaining normal functioning plus daily activities and/or exercising.

Caloric Balance

In order to . . .

Maintain Current Weight (or achieve a caloric balance): The daily intake of calories must be equivalent to the amount of calories burned each day.

Gain Body Fat (or achieve a positive caloric balance): The daily intake of calories must be greater than the amount of calories burned each day.

Lose Body Fat (or achieve a negative caloric balance): The daily intake of calories must be less than the amount of calories burned each day.

neither gaining nor losing weight. Unfortunately for Gary, he has recently been introduced to a new chocolate chip cookie recipe that he really likes. He makes a couple of batches of cookies each week and always has them on hand. Without even realizing it, Gary is now taking in about 200 more calories per day than his body needs. Caloric input is now at 2,700, and caloric output is still at 2,500. At this rate he will *gain 1 pound of body fat every 2.5 weeks* (3,500 calories per pound/200 extra calories per day = 17.5 days to gain 1 pound). Eventually, Gary's body will reach a point where it needs 200 extra calories a day to support the additional fat he has put on. He will then be at caloric balance again, with input and output each equaling 2,700 calories. He will also have 5 to 10 extra pounds of fat to support.

There are 3 ways input and output can be unbalanced to lose excess body fat:

(1) Reduce caloric intake below daily energy requirements,
(2) Maintain caloric intake and increase caloric output through additional physical activity above that included in the daily energy requirement,
(3) Combine 1 and 2 above to reduce caloric input *and* increase caloric output.

Let us assume that Gary, our hypothetical chocolate chip cookie lover, has decided to lose some weight. If he reduced his food intake from 2,700 calories to 2,200 calories per day, he would be 500 calories short of that required for him to maintain his current

FIGURE 3.1
Calorie Input and Gradual Weight Gain

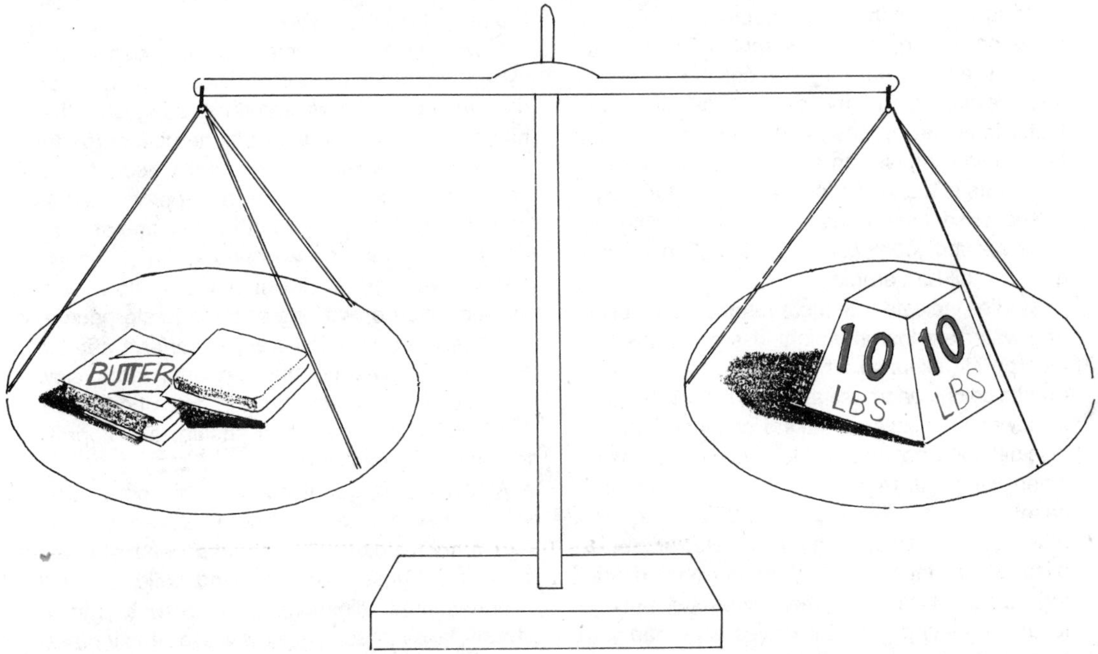

If a person were to consume one extra tablespoon of butter or margarine (100 calories) each day for one year, his or her theoretical weight gain would exceed 10 pounds.

weight. Since 1 pound of fat equals 3,500 calories, it would take Gary 7 days to lose 1 pound of fat (3,500/500 4eq 7). If, however, Gary decides to keep consuming 2,700 calories per day, he can still lose weight by increasing his energy need through exercise. If he starts a jogging program that burns an extra 250 calories per day, it will take about 2 weeks for him to lose 1 pound of fat, assuming he jogs every day (3,500/250 = 14). The best and most efficient way for Gary to lose his excess fat would be to decrease his caloric input and increase his caloric output. This would create a 750-calorie-per-day deficit or a weight loss of nearly 2 pounds per week (3,500/750 = 4.6). A less demanding regimen would have him exercise and cut his cookie consumption in half. Then he would lose 1 pound every 10 days (3,500/350 = 10) until caloric balance is once again achieved.

(continued on p. 49)

The Diet/Exercise Equation

WHY DIETS FAIL

In order to lose weight, the body must burn more calories than it consumes. Women, traditionally, focus on dieting, the "consumption" half of the formula, and all but forget about the "expenditure," exercise. But the single most important factor in achieving and maintaining ideal weight is aerobic exercise: an activity that can elevate heart rate to a specific level and keep it there for a sustained time period. Dancing, swimming, brisk walking, jogging, and cycling, if done properly, can all be aerobic.

Studies indicate that more fat and less muscle and water are lost in weight-loss programs that incorporate exercise. The body's response to a drastic caloric decrease and loss of lean tissue is a slower metabolism, making continued weight loss difficult if not impossible. The ultimate insult: when weight is regained (which is usually the case), it is more likely to be water and fat than muscle tissue resulting in an ever slower metabolism and a "fatter" body. Without exercise, dieting can produce a slimmer silhouette, but the failure of dieting is that it leaves a woman with the metabolism of a "fat" woman—a metabolism that will burn fewer calories.

The ideal weight-loss program combines judicious eating (*not* a starvation diet) with moderate aerobic exercise. Exercise burns body fat, speeds metabolism, and increases muscle tissue—which, in turn, burns more calories than fat burns.

EXERCISE BASICS

In designing a personal aerobic-exercise program, three essentials must be considered: exercise intensity, duration, and frequency.

Intensity refers to heart rate during exercise. Knowing correct exercise heart rate is the key to getting a proper aerobic workout. Research has shown that a heart rate representing 60 to 80 percent of maximum heart rate is aerobic and can increase cardiovascular capacity. Exercising below aerobic heart rate will not lead to a significant increase in stamina, and exercising above

your rate can be needlessly exhausting. Use the formula [on page 47] to establish your target (training) heart rate (THR).

Now that exercise intensity has been established, *duration* of workout sessions must be determined. Again, research has suggested that heart rate should be within its aerobic range for *at least twenty minutes* in order to benefit the cardiovascular system. The safe approach to this goal: taking five minutes both before and after an aerobic workout for a warm-up and a cool-down period. Warm up for five minutes by slowly jogging in place or walking at a moderate pace to get heart rate into THR range; perform aerobic exercise for twenty minutes; afterwards slow down for five minutes to bring down heart rate. The total workout session should take approximately thirty minutes.

A few words about duration: a woman who starts a new program may not be able to exercise for twenty minutes. She should do what she can without exhausting herself, and build up to a twenty-minute minimum. Don't rush to get in shape. Take it gradually, slowly, and keep it pleasant. The body will inevitably adapt to the stresses put on it, and a woman will be able to do more—more painlessly, too.

For women who would like to exercise longer than twenty minutes, that's O.K. In fact, the longer one exercises, the more the body relies on its fat stores for fuel. Over time, the body becomes more and more efficient at burning fat for fuel (instead of storing it on the hips). A poor reason to extend the length of an exercise session: to punish oneself for years of physical neglect. Positive reasons: genuine enjoyment and feelings of invigoration.

The *frequency* of aerobic sessions: at least three times a week in order to derive cardiovascular benefits. A woman may work out more frequently, but care should be taken to vary the intensity and/or the duration of the sessions. If one does a hard workout one day (e.g., 140 bpm for forty minutes), the next day should be easier

(120 bpm for thirty minutes) to allow the body time to recover.

The *type of activity* chosen for an aerobic workout should be one that elevates heart rate to the training zone, but also one that uses large muscle groups (legs, buttocks, arms) and that eventually can be sustained for thirty minutes or more. Walking briskly, jogging, swimming, cycling, rowing, and rope jumping are all excellent aerobic exercises; choose exercises that best suit your liking and environment. Alternating activities is a good way to keep up interest and to tone a variety of muscles.

Beginners: Obtain a physician's approval. Exercise at least three times a week at the low end of aerobic range. Aim to exercise for thirty minutes. You may need to start out at five minutes; take two to three weeks to build up.

EXERCISE GOAL: LONGER, NOT HARDER
An important point to remember is that for some women low-to-moderate heart rates (60–70 percent of maximum heart rate) may be more effective for burning body fat than higher heart rates. But if you decrease intensity, you should increase duration. Take a pleasant hike for one hour rather than an intense run for thirty minutes. Only competitive athletes need to train more intensely; to be slim and fit, exercise need not be painful or exhausting.

A good example of how working out too intensely may be counterproductive to weight-loss goals is the case of Annie, forty-one years old. She lost ten pounds in eight weeks by making small diet changes and riding her stationary bike five days a week for thirty to forty-five minutes at her *maximum* aerobic training rate (143 bpm). However, for several weeks she had not lost any more weight despite consistent cycling. When she consulted me, I asked her to keep her frequency (five times a week) and duration (thirty to forty-five minutes) constant, but to drop her heart rate ten to fifteen beats per minute to a *low-to-moderate* level (107–125 bpm). Following this new program, she lost eleven more pounds in two months. Annie thought harder was better and that a high heart rate would help her to lose weight faster.

Target Heart Rate

- **Estimated Maximum Heart Rate (HR max)** = 220 − your age (beats per minute)
- **Lower THR limit** = .60 × HR max (bpm)
- **Upper THR limit** = .80 × HR max (bpm)

E.g.: If you are 35 years old, training heart range is:

- **HR max** = 220 − 35 (= 185 bpm)
- **Appropriate aerobic training heart range:** between 111 (.60 × 185) bpm and 148 (.80 × 185) bpm.

In addition to helping a woman lose weight and body fat, aerobic exercise offers other benefits: Heart and lungs become more efficient; resting heart rate and blood pressure are lowered. Individuals report the quality of their sleep improves; moods become more even; feelings of well-being, confidence develop.

LOSING WEIGHT
Because most women think about weight loss in terms of cutting calories rather than burning them up, they opt for "starvation" diets that eventually fail them. A starvation diet is generally considered to be one that provides fewer than 800 calories per day. Drawbacks associated with a starvation diet include: reduced metabolic rate (and eventual failure to lose weight); loss of lean tissue (from muscles and organs); regaining of weight as fat and water (rather than lean tissue); malnutrition; and feelings of deprivation that can result in binging. By understanding the body's caloric needs and the number of calories that can be expended through aerobic exercise, women can learn how to lose weight without starving. A thirty-five year old, 130-pound woman's daily caloric expenditure may look like this:

Activity	Time	Calories Burned
Sleep	8 hrs.	300
Desk work	8 hrs.	620
Normal activities (e.g., cooking)	4 hrs.	360
Rest activities (e.g., reading)	4 hrs.	220
	24 hrs.	1500 cal/day

Most women mistakenly believe they cannot lose weight if they consume more than 1000 calories per day. This is not true. The reason: they neglect to take into account their weight and caloric needs. A look at this chart, for example, proves that our sample woman could lose a half pound of body fat every nine days by eating 1300 calories a day: a 200-calorie deficit each day over nine days adds up to 1800 calories, which is just over a half pound of body fat (one pound = 3500 calories). A diet of 1300 calories would supply this woman's energy and nutrition needs, maintain metabolic rate, prevent deprivation feelings.

A more effective and healthful weight-loss approach for our sample woman would be for her to decrease food intake *and* increase caloric expenditure through aerobic exercise in the following way:

• Consume 1400 calories/day, creating a 100-calorie deficit per day—or a 700-calorie deficit for one week.

• Exercise aerobically four days a week for thirty-five minutes—which burns approximately 110 extra calories for the week. (At 130 pounds, our exerciser burns about eight calories per minute at her training heart rate.)

• Through prudent diet *and* exercise, this woman can create an 1800-calorie deficit for the week—which equals about a half-pound loss of body fat.

HEALTHFUL EATING

A half-pound-to-one-pound weight loss per week may not sound like much when we're used to hearing about "diets" that promise losses of five to ten pounds each week. But when weight is lost through good nutrition combined with proper exercise, it not only makes a significant difference in appearance—but in a woman's stamina and health; because the weight lost is body *fat*, not lean tissue and water. Women should not be discouraged by what might seem like a slow rate of weight loss: The difference will be noticeable in how good one feels—and the losses are far more permanent.

Good nutrition, not dieting, is another important factor in attaining ideal weight. Eating a variety of wholesome foods not only assures a woman of getting basic nutrients but prevents her from developing cravings for foods high in fats and sugars. In general, the *ideal* diet has calories comprised of about 50–60 percent complex carbohydrates (grains, fruits, vegetables), less than 30 percent fats (oils, butter, margarine), and 10–20 percent protein (meat, fish, poultry, eggs). The basic American diet currently is about 46 percent carbohydrates, 43 percent fats, and 12–15 percent protein. Despite some gains, experts suggest we need to be more vegetarian-like: to substitute foods such as pasta, rice, breads, vegetables, and fruits for the large amounts of fat in our diets.

Along with maintaining a high standard for the foods we eat, a number of other techniques can help one lose weight and stay on a good eating plan over the long run.

1. Keep a food diary for two weeks. This will help you to become more aware of food habits and allow you to calculate daily caloric intake.

2. Never allow yourself to get very hungry. Research shows you will eat more if you delay eating past the time you feel hungry.

3. Eat frequently. A combination of small snacks and meals is ideal.

4. Don't skip meals.

5. Eat the majority of your daily calories during daytime hours, when you're active.

6. Eat slowly with taste, smell, and touch awareness.

7. Maintain a permissive attitude. "I can eat anything I want to; now, what do I *really* want to eat?"

8. There are no taboo foods, just taboo habits. Allow yourself small portions of "luxury" foods (e.g., desserts) from time to time.

9. Limit yourself to a maximum of two drinks three times per week.

10. After a binge, don't punish yourself the next day by starving; go back to normal eating.

TO START—AND KEEP IT UP

Make a few exercise and nutrition changes today, no matter how small, that you can incorporate into your life. If a change is not working for you, make adjustments. Don't make promises that, if you can't keep them, will propel you into abandoning the whole program. It's not how quickly you achieve a fitter, leaner self . . . but how long you maintain it.

Source: Julie Anthony, *Vogue* (July 1988), pp. 218–219, 248–249.

Weekly Exercise Program

Day	Activity	Intensity	Duration
Monday	Brisk walk	125 bpm	45 min.
Tuesday	Stationary bike	140 bpm	30 min.
Wednesday	Rest		
Thursday	Aerobic dance	135 bpm	30 min.
Friday	Brisk walk	115 bpm	40 min.
Saturday	Rest		
Sunday	Walk/jog	140 bpm	30 min.

EXERCISE AND WEIGHT LOSS

Although it is true that one can achieve a negative caloric balance either by restricting diet or by exercising, the best plans for weight reduction call for a balance of both. The value of exercise for weight reduction seems to be underestimated. For example, many popular diet programs lack information concerning exercise. Exercising while on a calorie-restricting diet will increase the rate of weight loss without jeopardizing health. Some weight-loss plans that don't include exercise might even impair health. Exercise can lessen one's appetite and allow for greater flexibility in diet. In this case, those having a difficult time adhering to a restrictive diet can exercise to compensate for the excess calories they may be consuming. Exercise temporarily raises the metabolic rate, and, in relation to the setpoint theory previously discussed, exercise may help to keep the metabolic rate from dropping during caloric restriction and assist in establishing a new setpoint for body fat. [1] Finally, combining exercise with diet protects against the loss of lean muscle tissue, which so often happens when weight loss is achieved by diet alone.

The preservation of lean tissue mass is partly due to aerobic exercise training that enhances the mobilization and break-

(continued on p. 51)

FIGURE 3.2
Fat Digestion

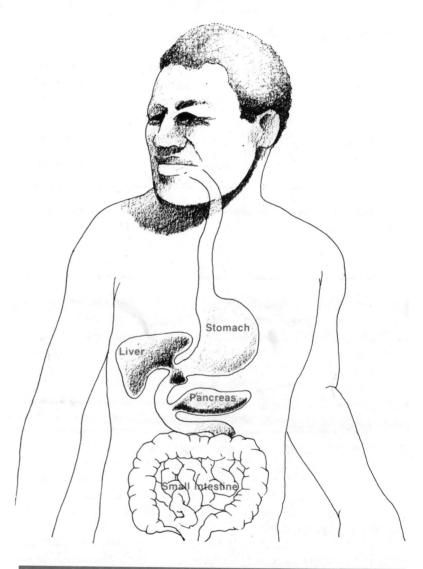

When food is ingested, fat is separated from the other food elements in the stomach
and enters the small intestine where it is broken down and absorbed into the
bloodstream. The fat is then either burned as energy or stored in the body's fat
deposits. If the fat is not absorbed, it continues on its way and is excreted.

down of fat from the body's adipose deposits. In addition, vigorous exercise tends to increase the rate of protein buildup in
skeletal muscle, while at the same time retarding its rate of
breakdown. This protein-sparing effect causes a greater portion
of the caloric deficit to be made up by the breakdown of fat. [2]

Exercise Myths

Misconceptions about exercise abound and may keep some obese
people from initiating or maintaining an exercise program. It is
important to examine and dispel these beliefs if exercise is to take
its rightful place in healthy weight-loss programs.

Myth #1: Increased activity causes a subsequent increase in
appetite that would contribute to a weight problem. This is
simply not true. Exercise helps to stimulate the appetite-control
mechanisms so that excessive calories are less likely to be consumed. It is in sedentary people that the appetite-control mechanism does not function properly.

Myth #2: Exercise really does not burn enough calories to
make any significant difference in weight loss. Those not inclined
to exercise often present statistics indicating that extreme
amounts of exercise are needed to lose significant amounts of
body fat. For example, it has been cited that "one must chop wood
for 10 hours, golf for 20 hours, perform mild calisthenic exercises
for 22 hours, or play ping pong for 28 hours or volleyball for 32
hours, or run 35 miles just to reduce body fat by 1 pound." [3]
While these numbers may be accurate, they do not represent the
typical way exercise is used in a weight-reduction program.
Experts neither expect nor recommend that people exercise to the
extent that they would lose a pound of fat a day. The recommendation for safe and effective long-term weight loss is 1 to 2 pounds
per week. Given that the effects of exercise are cumulative, it is
not unrealistic to think that a person could lose 1 pound through
a moderate exercise program over a period of 7 to 14 days. An
even better way to look at exercise is over a longer period of time.
If a 125-pound woman were to walk 1 hour a day at a moderate
pace (3 miles/hour) 4 days per week for a year, the theoretical
weight loss would be nearly 12 pounds. In addition to the pounds
lost, exercise would provide this individual with greater appetite
control, improved body tone, and, depending on the type of
exercise, numerous benefits for the heart, lungs, and circulatory
system.

Another way to demonstrate the importance of exercise in
weight-reduction programs is to look at recommended caloric
allowances. Caloric recommendations for sedentary men are usu-

(continued on p. 54)

Did You Know That . . .

A California nutritionist has her patients wear pedome-
ters to measure how far they walk.
Obese women find they normally
walk only half as much as those
of normal weight.

Several years ago, J. P. Flatt, a professor of biochemistry at the University of Massachusetts Medical School in Worcester, put a laboratory mouse in a cage with an exercise wheel and gave the mouse access to as much food as it cared to eat. In return for this cushy life style, the mouse had to submit to daily metabolic measurements.

At first, the mouse ignored the exercise wheel. Then one day it began running and soon was spinning the wheel at a rate of nearly 40,000 turns a day. The mouse's appetite quickly fell off and it began to lose weight, getting the higher levels of energy needed to sustain the running by utilizing its fat. Then, after two weeks of running, the mouse began to eat again. In fact, its appetite was even more robust than before, because it was eating enough to meet the increased energy needs brought on by its new life as a dedicated runner.

Balancing the Equation of Fat and Exercise

The result, as Flatt recounted it in a paper [in 1987], was a mouse trim and able to eat more than before without gaining weight. . . . [T]he mouse had achieved a new metabolic steady state.

In a society concerned about fat and the quest for fitness, the moral is that exercise can be the key to weight loss and a trimmer body. But to Flatt, who has spent his career studying diet, obesity and metabolism—or how food is converted into energy by the body—in both mice and men, the significance of the running mouse is more subtle.

Flatt is a leading theorist in the world of diet, fat and metabolism. The metabolic steady state is central to his ideas about why we become fat and why we lose weight, through dieting or exercise.

He argues that if we eat too much fat it makes us plump, which is not a revolutionary idea in itself. Nutritionists have long said that because fat has more calories per gram than carbohydrates, fat provides extra calories that cause us to gain weight. To cut back on total calories, they advise, eat less fat.

Flatt contends that the system is much more complex than that. If you merely want to maintain your present weight, eat less fat. But he further proposes that the ability to lose weight is governed by the relative amounts of fats and carbohydrates that we eat.

During digestion, carbohydrates are converted to **glucose**, which goes directly to the cells to provide energy. Excess glucose is stored as **glycogen**. Because in modern society we have plenty of carbohydrates to eat, glycogen stores are always high and any extra fat in the diet quickly becomes fat on the body. Therefore if you want to lose weight, he says, you must cut down on your total food intake. This will naturally lead to fewer carbohydrates and lowered glycogen stores. This will then increase the body's ability to burn fat through a mechanism that is as yet unknown.

Glucose: A monosaccharide or simple sugar found in foods by itself and also as part of complex carbohydrates and the disaccharides sucrose, maltose, and lactose; also known as blood sugar.

Glycogen: A form of complex carbohydrate stored in the body. It is found primarily in liver and muscle tissue.

Flatt's ideas, which are far from proven, are important because they provide a new way of looking at diet and exercise. The advice, cut down on fats, may be familiar, but new insight into what is going on in the body if we reduce fats is likely to provide better ways of using diet and exercise to control weight problems.

Although Flatt began to form his ideas a decade ago, it has only been in the last year or two that studies of both animals and humans have begun to bear him out.

"I am unaware of anyone trying to disprove my ideas, but I don't think they have gained wide acceptance yet," he said recently. "On the other hand, I don't think it is that there are many arguments made against it."

The core of the Flatt fat doctrine comes from studies in which mice were given as much to eat as they wanted of diets that had varying amounts of fat and carbohydrates. As expected, the mice who ate high-fat diets grew obese. But when the scientists studied what was happening to the mice from a metabolic standpoint, the picture was more complex.

If one is to maintain a constant weight, or metabolic steady state, the energy being used by the cells should directly reflect the energy present in the food. Thus, if the amount of fats and carbohydrates in the diet are equal, the fuel going to the cells to provide energy should come half from fat in the diet and half from carbohydrates.

But the mouse experiments found that the amount of fat being used to provide fuel for the body was relatively constant, regardless of how much fat was being eaten. The mice eating a diet with 64 percent fat, an enormous amount of fat by human standards, used only a small part of this fat initially to fuel the body. The rest was stored as fat. The ultra high-fat cage was quickly filled with mice who waddled.

Eventually, however, the mice grew fat enough so that the body's metabolism began to shift. The proportion of fat and carbohydrate being burned as fuel in the cells began to directly reflect the amount present in the food. The body had reached a new steady state, albeit a very fat steady state related to a fat-rich diet.

Flatt has proposed that humans have metabolic systems that behave in the same way. If we are eating far more fat than the body needs on a daily basis, the fat is stored and our clothes soon become tight. Eventually, we reach a new steady state in which we are fat but gain no additional weight. The unnecessary fat in the daily diet is now being burned by the cells to meet our daily energy requirements.

According to Flatt's theory, if we constantly eat so much that our glycogen stores are always full, excessive amounts of fat in the diet will not be burned until we reach a fatter steady state. If we begin dieting and keep the glycogen stores at a lower level, the body will begin turning to fat in the diet and stored fat to meet its energy needs.

After years of studying diet, fat and exercise, Flatt has come to see the metabolic world in terms of the body's burning, or oxidation, of fat. The burning of fat can be promoted in three ways.

Did You Know That . . .

Few of our Stone Age ancestors were obese: they ate less fat (wild game is leaner than domesticated animals) and sodium than we do, and 5 to 10 times more fiber (from wild plants).

The first, and least desirable, is to grow fat enough so that all the fat in the diet is used to maintain the body's steady state, rather than add new fat. Another is to restrict what you eat so that glycogen stores are always somewhat depleted and the body must turn to fat to meet its needs. A third is aerobic exercise.

Ultimately, the body must burn as much fat and carbohydrate each day as it takes in as food if the body's overall weight and the fat padding it are to remain constant.

Fat in our food has already been indicted in connection with development of heart disease. If Flatt is right that the proportion of fat in the diet is just as important as how much we eat over all in terms of maintaining a lean body, then we have an extra incentive to pass up the next bowl of ice cream and settle for another serving of pasta—without the sauce, of course.

Source: William Stockton, *New York Times*, 12 December 1988, sec. 3, pp. 11–12.

ally around 2,400 calories per day, while the recommendations for very active men, such as lumberjacks and highly trained athletes, range from 4,500 to 6,000 calories per day. Certainly no weight-reduction program should exclude any factor that can more than double caloric requirements. While an intense 4,500 to 6,000 calorie-per-day exercise regimen is not recommended for the average person, much less an overweight, previously sedentary person, the effects of a 100- to 200-calorie-per-day exercise program can prove significant over time. Remember, however, that although exercise has many positive benefits, it cannot do everything.

Myth #3: One can selectively reduce overly fat areas of the body by **spot reduction**, or selectively exercising that area of the body. In other words, if one is fat in the thighs, then exercises for the thighs will solve the problem. While this is an attractive idea for those who have excessive fat stores in one particular area of the body, it simply is not true. Spot reduction exercise will improve the tension and strength of underlying muscle tissue and cause generalized fat reduction over the entire body, but it will not cause fat to be lost from just one area of the body.

An experiment conducted at the University of Massachusetts, Amherst, which tested the idea of spot reduction, bears this out. Thirteen men performed 5,004 sit-ups during a 27-day period. Prior to the exercise, samples of fat tissue were taken from the abdomen, buttocks, and shoulder area. If the spot reduction theory were correct, then the fat cells in the abdominal area would have been reduced in size while the other areas remained unchanged or changed less significantly. The results of

Spot reduction: The unfounded belief that exercising selected areas of the body will result in a greater loss of excess fat in that area than would otherwise occur as a result of whole-body exercise.

Table 3.1
"I Can Walk It Off": Minutes of Exercise Needed to Burn Up Some Common Foods*

Walking	Bicycling	Swimming	Running	Burns up roughly . . .
19 min	12 min	9 min	5 min	**100 calories:** 1 apple or 2 strips bacon or 1 glass beer or 1 glass soda or 1 oz cheddar cheese or 1 fried egg or 1 glass orange juice or 1 pancake (with syrup) or 10 potato chips
38 min	24 min	18 min	10 min	**200 calories:** 1/2 cup cereal (with milk and sugar) or 1/2 breast fried chicken or 1/4 lb halibut steak or 1/6 quart ice cream or 1 10-oz glass whole milk or 1 slice pizza
57 min	36 min	27 min	15 min	**300 calories:** 1 loin pork chop or 2 doughnuts or 1 tuna fish sandwich or 1/3 quart ice milk
77 min	49 min	36 min	21 min	**400 calories:** 1 milk shake or 1 piece apple pie or 1 roast beef sandwich (with gravy) or 1 piece strawberry shortcake

*Calories expended by a 154-lb person. Walking briskly (at 3 1/2 mph) uses up about 5 calories per minute; riding a bicycle, 8 calories per minute; swimming, 11 calories per minute; and running, 19 calories per minute.
Source: George A. Bray, M.D., *The Obese Patient* (New York: W. B. Saunders, 1976).

the study indicated no difference in fat cell size for any of the 3 areas. [4]

This summary capsulizes the idea of spot reduction in a concise and understandable manner:

> There is widespread belief that by exercising one area of the body, more fat will be lost from that area in comparison to other body parts. It is also believed that disuse of a muscle group causes a disproportionate accumulation of local **subcutaneous** fat, and, conversely, [that] an increase in a muscle activity facilitates a relatively large fat mobilization from the specific storage sites. While the notion of "spot reduction" through selective exercises such as leg raises, sit-ups, side bends, or trunk twists is especially attractive from an aesthetic standpoint (and monetarily to those who peddle special creams, shakers and rollers), the scientific evidence does not support such practices. [5]

Myth #4: Exercise causes one to gain weight. In some respects this is actually true. Exercise causes one to lose fat and also to increase lean muscle tissue. Since muscle tissue weighs more than fat, it is possible that one could actually gain weight as the result of a successful exercise program. It is important to consider that the ultimate goal of a weight-loss program is to become

Subcutaneous: Beneath the skin, as in a subcutaneous injection.

(continued on p. 58)

Ever wonder how many calories a cookie contains? One typical cookie contains around 80 calories, meaning that an innocent snack of six chocolate chip cookies and a glass of milk probably has at least 600 calories, depending on how full of chocolate and nuts the cookies are. A middle-aged male who is 6 feet and 180 pounds probably needs around 2,500 calories a day to meet his nutritional needs without gaining weight.

When Exercise Isn't Enough

So, the simple snack has accounted for one-quarter of what he should eat that day.

Which brings us to the subject of fitness and weight control.

For most sedentary people, and particularly for those in their middle years, getting into shape usually encompasses a desire to lose some weight, perhaps 10 pounds; in some cases, 20 pounds or more. The painful truth is this: If you want to lose weight, it doesn't matter how much you exercise if you don't begin paying attention to how much and what you eat. You cannot consume 3,000 or 4,000 calories a day on a routine basis and expect exercise to lead to weight loss.

The first step, according to weight-loss experts, is to find out how much you are eating and what is accounting for the calories. You must do this carefully and honestly before you deny yourself the first mouthful.

"Most people have little idea how much they are eating," said Dr. Loren Greene, an endocrinologist and assistant clinical professor at New York University. She specializes in treating obesity.

Begin by purchasing a paperback book that lists the caloric content of foods. These books list foods both generically and by brand name and give the caloric content of typical servings. Spend some time looking at the book. It will be a real eye-opener.

Did you know that a handful of peanuts contains 160 calories? Or that a glass of wine or a soft drink contains 100 calories? On the other hand, a rice cake contains only 35 calories and mustard is essentially calorie-free. An apple has 61 calories and one-third cup of Kellogg's All Bran, eaten dry, has 70 calories.

As these truths begin to sink in, take the next step. Buy an inexpensive kitchen scale and begin keeping track of what you eat every day, right down to the sugar in the coffee at work. Do it for several days, and total up the caloric intake each day.

Armed with this self-awareness you are ready to begin changing your dietary life style. Make no mistake, just as getting fit and staying fit requires a commitment that must last a lifetime, getting down to ideal weight and staying there requires the same singlemindedness. For most people, losing the weight is not merely a matter of cutting down on the amount of foods eaten, it also means changing many of the foods.

For example, one gram of fat contains more calories than one gram

Do You Know How Much You're Eating?

Food	Serving size	Calories
Spaghetti (al dente)	1 cup	216
Spinach (boiled)	1/2 cup	18
Swordfish steak (broiled)	3" × 3" × 1/2"	218
Yogurt (plain, low-fat)	8 ounces	110
Apple (with skin)	2 1/2 diameter	61
Raw carrot	5 1/2 × 1/2"	21
Chocolate cupcake	1 cupcake	170
McDonald's Big Mac	1 hamburger	570
Dry roasted peanuts	1 ounce	160
Peanut butter	1 tablespoon	108
Domino's pizza (double cheese, pepperoni)	1 slice, 16" pie	389

Source: Barbara Kraus, *Calorie Guide to Brand Names & Basic Foods* (Signet Books, 1988).

of carbohydrate. The more you shift your diet away from fats to carbohydrates, the better off you are from a caloric standpoint. (You are also likely to be better off from a heart-disease standpoint, too.) So cut out, or at least cut down on, things like nuts, whole milk, chocolate, cookies, fried snack foods, potato chips, french fries, steaks, hamburgers, ham and cheese sandwiches and milkshakes.

Cut out sugar wherever you can. For example, drink only artificially sweetened soft drinks. Better yet, switch to seltzer, which has no salt, and flavor it with a slice of lime. Search out the low-fat milk, cheeses and yogurts. Study the nutritional information on cereal boxes for those that aren't sweetened and are low in fat.

Cooked pasta makes an excellent calorie-reducing meal, but you defeat its virtues if a rich, fatty sauce is poured over the pasta when it is served. There are tasty, low-calorie, low-fat sauces on the market that can liven up pasta.

Unbuttered popcorn is a low-calorie snack. So are rice cakes. Raw vegetables—carrots, cauliflower, broccoli—are excellent.

With your book, become an expert on the caloric content of foods. Become fanatical about seeking out low-calorie, low-fat nutritious foods. And then shift your diet toward them, remembering to maintain a balanced diet in the process.

Find out from a dietitian, a doctor, or a reputable nutrition book how many calories someone of your age and build needs on a daily basis. Pick a total daily intake that is only slightly below this target. A weight loss of a half pound or one pound a week is a realistic goal. A typical mistake is to try to do too much at once, just as some people begin exercising too strenuously at first.

As you change your diet, continue to count up each day how many calories you consume, and if you do go over one day, recognize that you will immediately have to make up the deficit the next day. You cannot sustain your dieting if you indulge in this sort of eating several days in a row.

Moreover, you must recognize that someone can eat too much of a low-calorie food. "You can gain weight on anything if you eat enough of it," Greene warned, telling of a patient who switched to popcorn as a weight-control measure but then ate so much that she continued to gain weight.

Unfortunately, this dietary regimen is boring. Fats and sugar add taste to foods, which is why pecan pie is more appealing than a raw carrot. And this new way of eating is not a short-term project that will end in a few weeks. You are facing a lifetime dietary change.

But once aerobic workouts and sensible eating are combined, the results in three months or so can be miraculous. If you are eating just enough to meet your daily nutritional requirements, the calories consumed in the aerobic workouts are likely to be translated into weight loss, provided you maintain discipline at the dinner table. If you are trying to maintain your current weight, 1,000 calories of exercise a week means you can eat 1,000 calories more.

And here is an added bonus: There is growing evidence that the aerobically fit body burns more fat than the body that is not fit, which can further help in weight reduction.

But the key ingredient in both becoming aerobically fit and losing weight has to come from within. You must commit to changing your life style if the results you achieve are to last more than a few months.

Source: William Stockton, *New York Times*, 20 February 1989, sec. 3, p. 11.

leaner, not necessarily lighter. This is especially important for a person only slightly overweight. Even though one may weigh more, the composition of the body has been altered favorably. Before the exercise program, the individual looked fat; now he or she looks trim and fit. The ultimate proof of successful weight reduction should not be on the bathroom scales, but in the bedroom mirror.

Getting Started with Exercise

Before beginning any exercise program, it is important to obtain medical clearance from a physician. This is particularly important for all people over 30 years of age who have been sedentary for a period of time and for all severely obese persons, regardless of age. During the medical examination, it is important to discuss with the physician the proposed exercise program. If there are medical conditions that would counter-indicate such activity, they should be detected here. For example, persons with high blood

(continued on p. 62)

FIGURE 3.3
The Spot Reduction Myth

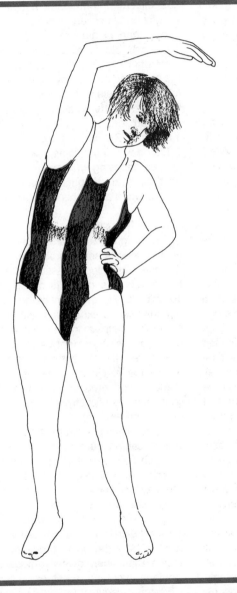

The spot reduction myth says that selectively exercising a particular area ("spot") of the body will result in a loss of fat in that area, the thighs for example. Research has conclusively demonstrated, however, that this is not true. While exercise is always valuable, no exercise will cause fat to be lost from just one area of the body.

Safe Exercise for the Overweight

The advertisements for exercise clothing and fitness classes would have you believe that physical activity is exclusively pursued by people with beautiful bodies for the sole purpose of keeping them that way. For years this image of exercise only for the already trim has kept millions of overweight people off running trails and bicycles and out of sweats and swimsuits.

But now there is a new fitness craze in the making, and its practitioners are all at least 30 percent above the "ideal" body weight—by definition, obese. Their primary goals are improved health and well-being, not necessarily weight control. Most of the practitioners are women, and many have ridden the weight-loss, weight-gain seesaw for years and now want off.

In their pursuit of physical activity, they are seeking physiques that are leaner and stronger, self-images that are sounder and bodies that are more resistant to ailment and accident. They want to increase their stamina and feel good about themselves and the bigger-than-average body.

As Pat Lyons and Debby Burgard put it in their newly published book, "Great Shape: The First Exercise Guide for Large Women" (Arbor House), "We have found that some of the miseries we attributed to our weight were in fact miseries of lives without movement, lives without play, lives without deep breathing and zest."

For many big women and men, embarrassment about their size, painful memories of childhood taunts, humiliations suffered as adults and the simple lack of exercise clothes that fit have long kept them confined to the couch instead of smashing tennis balls or swimming laps.

Now a growing number of exercise classes that cater to the special needs of overweight people, along with a growing industry that permits them to dress fashionably and comfortably for workouts, has prompted many to abandon the sedentary life that aggravated their weight problems.

Their efforts are well-timed. Recent research has indicated that many people with lifelong weight problems are more the victims of their genes than of gluttony and laziness, and that undefined biochemical factors seem to doom their efforts at weight reduction. Furthermore, the body has been shown to protect itself against low-calorie diets by reducing the number of calories it uses. After years of yo-yo dieting, people may find that they gain weight on as little as 1,000 to 1,500 calories a day.

Faced with these facts, many overweight people are choosing wellness rather than slimness as their goal, although a modest reduction in girth is often a side benefit of increased activity.

The Health Benefits

Overweight people are especially prone to a host of serious health problems, including heart disease, high blood pressure, diabetes and arthritis. Exercise counters all of these. Regular aerobic activity that can be sustained for long periods without exhaustion, like brisk walking or swimming, helps to lower the harmful blood fats, LDL-choelsterol and triglycerides, and raises the protective HDL-cholesterol. Exercise also improves the efficiency of the heart and helps to reduce blood pressure, normalize blood sugar, keep joints mobile, strengthen bones and relieve depression and anxiety.

Unlike dieting, exercise can permanently increase caloric burn by replacing metabolically sluggish body fat with metabolically active lean muscle tissue. Thus, a physically active fat person may lose some weight without having to diet. Even more weight can be lost when exercise is coupled with a modest reduction in calories that does not disrupt the normal metabolic rate—say, 200 to 500 a day. In fact, several studies have shown that when overweight people exercise regularly they tend to eat less.

Exercise also whittles away inches, even without weight loss, as muscle tissue replaces fat and muscle tone improves. And when combined with a weight-reducing diet, physical activity can prevent the loss of lean muscle tissue (including heart muscle) that occurs when diet alone is used to lose weight. When dieting without exercise, one-quarter to one-half the weight lost is muscle, not fat.

Psychological benefits can be even more dramatic, according to the authors of "Great Shape," who themselves are overweight. Ms Lyons, a registered nurse, said: "I found I loved physical activity for the ability it gave me to do something challenging and wonderful spontaneously. I became healthier not only by becoming more physically active but also by learning to integrate my mind, spirit and emotions into activity."

The authors quote Lee Eastman of Cornelius, Ore., who said, "I feel capable, more self-confident and assured and find myself doing things that in the past I would have waited for my husband to do for me." Since beginning an exercise program, she has become a dance exercise instructor for large women.

Many overweight people also find that adopting a regular exercise program encourages them to improve their eating habits. As Mrs. Eastman said: "It hit me one day that I was working so hard to get my body healthy I should pay attention to its nutritional needs as well. "I've cut down on salt and fat and have increased my fiber intake and am aware of my calcium levels."

Adapting Exercise Programs

An overweight person cannot simply flip on a Jane Fonda tape and zip through the routines without risk. Jeannette V. Harris, a registered dietitian who is a nutrition counselor in New York City, says these factors should be considered in designing safe and effective exercise programs.

• **Health status.** An obese person of any age should have a medical checkup for possible health risks before undertaking an exercise program. Ms. Harris suggests taking girth measurements (but not weight) so that exercise-related improvements can be readily detected.

• **Body shape.** Exercises that compress the chest cavity may impair breathing in those with excessive upper-body weight. Routines that require bending at the waist or hanging down should be avoided or modified.

• **Orthopedic problems.** All exercise should be done on a cushioned surface in well-padded shoes appropriate for the activity. The exercise routine should be low-impact (toes stay on the floor) to minimize stress on the back and legs. Many specialists promote swimming and water aerobics as ideal low-risk activities for people who are significantly overweight.

• **Exercise intensity.** Some overweight people are too out of condition to begin with aerobic activities. They should start with stretching and strengthening exercises. Aerobic activities for those who are overweight should begin at moderate intensity, with a pulse rate from 60 to 75 percent of maximum aerobic capacity. This range is determined by subtracting your age from the number 220 and then multiplying the result by 0.60 for the lowest pulse rate and 0.75 for the highest rate to be reached in exercise. Once conditioned to this level of exercise, the intensity can be gradually increased to a maximum of 85 percent of aerobic capacity.

• **Heat intolerance.** Overweight people often sweat heavily and get overheated even with minimum exertion. In warm weather, exercise is best done in a well-ventilated or air-conditioned area. Loose, light clothing should be worn. The pulse rate should be checked often to avoid overexertion and lots of water should be consumed before, during and after the activity.

• **Poor self-image.** To combat self-consciousness and intimidating self-comparisons with thinner participants, exercise classes should be limited to people with similar weight problems, preferably with an instructor who is also large. The class atmosphere should be instructive, supportive and noncompetitive, with each participant encouraged to do only what he or she can handle comfortably.

• **Body awareness.** Many overweight people, accustomed to living from the neck up, tend to ignore signals of distress from the lower body. But, while exercising, it is important to realize that symptoms like breathing difficulties, chest or muscle pain and weakness are warnings to slow down, modify or stop the activity.

To locate exercise programs intended for overweight people, check the advertisements in magazines like *Radiance* and *Big Beautiful Woman* or get in touch with stores that sell clothing for large people.

In some areas, local Y's or health clubs offer dance-exercise or water aerobics classes that are suitable. Women at Large of Yakima, Wash., has franchised 26 fitness salons throughout the country and in Canada. You can also consult the appendix of "Great Shape," which lists clothing suppliers and videos intended for large women, as well as exercise programs throughout the country.

Source: Jane Brody, "Personal Health," *New York Times,* 8 September 1988, sec. 2, p. 12.

pressure should not engage in **isometric exercises** that involve pushing or pulling against an immovable object. This type of exercise tends to raise blood pressure considerably. Persons with joint problems should probably look for activities other than jogging or aerobic dance because these activities can be hard on the joints. There are no physical limitations, however, that should preclude participation in an exercise program of some sort. Even people who are classified as "high risk" can exercise. Their programs need to be individually tailored to their needs and supervised by trained medical personnel.

Once cleared by a physician to undertake an exercise program, the next step is to decide upon an appropriate form of exercise. It is important that the exercise be of sufficient frequency, intensity, and duration to create the desired weight loss and to improve other aspects of health as well.

The actual type of exercise chosen is important. It should be an exercise that is enjoyable and preferably one that will improve the condition of one's cardiovascular system as well as produce weight loss. Traditionally, activities such as jogging, swimming, aerobic dance, and bicycling have been recommended. These are all excellent choices, although some evidence exists that swimming is less effective in reducing body fat than the other activities in this group. Competitive sports, such as handball, racquetball, tennis, and basketball, can also prove effective for weight loss and cardiovascular fitness if done regularly and at sufficient intensity. The problem with these activities is that they require one or more other people to participate, a court or special surface to play on, and, generally, more time than do individual activities. It should also be noted that one need not limit oneself to a single activity. It is now popular to "cross train," to combine several different activities in a program. This may increase the fun of exercising and reduce the boredom that often results in abandoning programs.

Another activity that is gaining in popularity is walking. There are many advantages to walking. It is virtually injury-free, has a low drop-out rate, requires no special skill, and can be done

Isometric exercise: An exercise in which a muscle or set of muscles is pitted against either an immovable object or another muscle or set of muscles.

(continued on p. 64)

FIGURE 3.4
Walking and Weight Loss

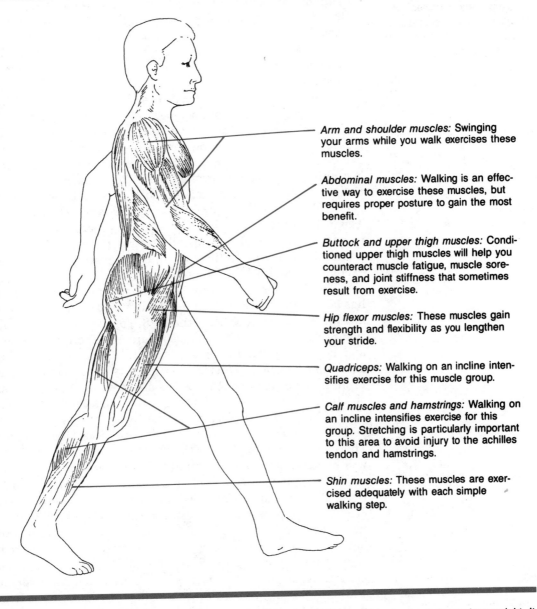

Arm and shoulder muscles: Swinging your arms while you walk exercises these muscles.

Abdominal muscles: Walking is an effective way to exercise these muscles, but requires proper posture to gain the most benefit.

Buttock and upper thigh muscles: Conditioned upper thigh muscles will help you counteract muscle fatigue, muscle soreness, and joint stiffness that sometimes result from exercise.

Hip flexor muscles: These muscles gain strength and flexibility as you lengthen your stride.

Quadriceps: Walking on an incline intensifies exercise for this muscle group.

Calf muscles and hamstrings: Walking on an incline intensifies exercise for this group. Stretching is particularly important to this area to avoid injury to the achilles tendon and hamstrings.

Shin muscles: These muscles are exercised adequately with each simple walking step.

Walking will shape and tone muscles in the abdomen, buttocks, hips, and legs, and can also help you lose weight. It requires no special skills, can be done anywhere and anytime, and is virtually free of any risk of injury.

almost anywhere and anytime. Research also indicates that walking can be an effective aid in weight loss. In one study, those who used diet alone lost 7 pounds, those who walked and did not diet lost 6 pounds, and those who combined diet and walking lost 13 pounds. At both the 8- and 24-week follow-ups, the diet and walking group continued to lose weight, while the other two groups did not. [6]

An additional factor in selecting the right exercise is the frequency with which one can perform that exercise. From the cardiovascular perspective, research has shown that 3 to 4 times per week is the minimum needed to obtain desired benefits. [7] From a weight-reduction perspective, the more exercise, the better. This does not mean that one must exercise even when feeling tired or ill. It must be remembered, however, that forgoing exercise means a less favorable caloric balance for that day. In the beginning of a program, it might be better to exercise only 3 to 4 times a week and then gradually build up to perhaps 5 to 6 times per week. This will help prevent injuries and extreme fatigue. The most important aspect of an exercise program is the motivation to continue, and nothing will destroy motivation faster than a chronic injury or feelings of total exhaustion brought on by exercising too much or too quickly.

The duration of the exercise is another important factor. It has been established that 20 to 30 minutes per day is an optimal amount for cardiovascular fitness. [8] For weight loss, the duration of the exercise will vary depending on the type of exercise and how many calories one wishes to burn. See table 3.2 to determine how many calories each activity burns per 30 minutes. From this, one can make decisions about how long to exercise to obtain the desired results. There are, of course, individual differences. While two people may do the same activity for the same period of time, one may burn more calories than the other. Therefore, an adjustment in the duration of the exercise routine will be necessary to suit individual needs.

The final factor related to exercise selection is intensity. Intensity refers to how hard one works during the exercise period. Traditionally, people believed that one could obtain optimal benefit by exercising at 60 percent of capacity, but more recent studies have indicated that levels as low as 45 percent can produce significant improvements. [9] What does this mean to the average person? As a general rule, if you can carry on a conversation while exercising, you are probably okay. If you are experiencing difficulty breathing or talking, you are pushing yourself too much and should exercise at a more manageable level.

Table 3.2 Exercising to Lose Weight

Swimming (20 yd/min)	145 calories*
Walking (4 mph)	175 calories
Aerobics (low-impact)	205 calories
Calisthenic circuit training	270 calories
Jogging (5 mph)	270 calories
Aerobics (high-impact)	280 calories
Bicycling (13 mph)	320 calories
Swimming (55 yd/min)	395 calories
Rowing	435 calories
Cross-country skiing (8 mph)	470 calories
Running (8 mph)	470 calories

*Note: Estimated calories burned in 30 minutes by a 150-pound person.

Source: *Consumer Reports Health Letter,* February 1990.

Any physical activity burns calories, but some burn more than others. Listed above are the calories burned in 30 minutes by a 150-pound person who engages in a variety of common exercise activities. Persons weighing less than 150 pounds will burn fewer calories than shown; those weighing over 150 pounds will burn more.

In addition to a planned exercise program, one can also increase activity levels by making small changes in one's daily life-style, for example: parking the car at the far end of the lot; walking up steps instead of taking the elevator; walking 10 minutes instead of taking a coffee break; using a push-type lawn mower instead of a riding mower; and so on. These ideas may sound strange to the average American, who believes that convenience is best. It may be a good idea, for the sake of good health, to try to use more energy—and get more exercise.

One can lose weight by increasing caloric output (exercising), by decreasing caloric input (dieting), or by a combination of both. Research clearly indicates that the best way is by combining diet and exercise.

In order to encourage people to make exercise an important component in their weight-control programs, it is often necessary to dispel myths regarding exercise. Such statements often come from people who do not understand exercise and probably have little desire to try it. They use these myths as excuses. If they were to forget the myths and start to exercise, they would no doubt find the results rewarding. W

4

Weight Control, Diet, and Behavior Modification

I
T HAS BEEN ESTIMATED that in America one-half of the women and one-quarter of the men have at some time reduced their food intake to lose weight. Sixteen percent of American women say they are continually on a diet. Artificial sweetener sales have doubled in the last decade, while expenditures for over-the-counter diet aids reached $228 million and expenditures for low-calorie foods soared to $7 billion. [1] There is no question that America is a weight-conscious, diet-oriented society.

DIET

Diet is the most visible aspect of weight-control programs. Properly used, the word **diet** refers to a person's ordinary day-by-day consumption of food and drink. It would be more correct here to use the phrase **weight-loss diet** when referring to the narrower concept of following a restricted plan of food and drink consumption in order to meet a specific individual goal to lose body fat. However, for simplicity's sake, here the term "diet" refers to restricted caloric intake unless otherwise noted.

Although there are literally hundreds of diets available to choose from, many are unhealthy and should be avoided. The secret to developing, preparing, and maintaining an effective weight-control diet is really no secret at all. The two key ele-

Diet: A person's ordinary and customary daily consumption of food and drink.

Weight-loss diet: A plan of food and drink consumption followed in order to meet a specific weight-loss goal.

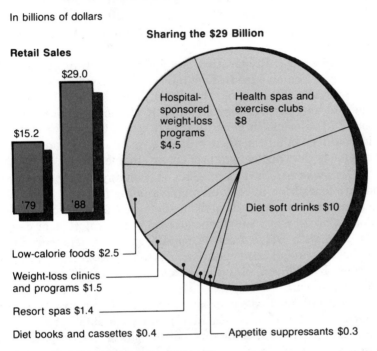

FIGURE 4.1
The American Diet Market

In billions of dollars

Sharing the $29 Billion

Retail Sales

$29.0

$15.2

'79   '88

Hospital-sponsored weight-loss programs $4.5

Health spas and exercise clubs $8

Diet soft drinks $10

Low-calorie foods $2.5

Weight-loss clinics and programs $1.5

Resort spas $1.4

Diet books and cassettes $0.4

Appetite suppressants $0.3

Source: *New York Times,* 26 November 1989, p. 17.

The diet-help industry has grown increasingly lucrative since the late 1970s: Its profits almost doubled between 1979 and 1988.

ments, nutrient balance and caloric restriction, are clearly understood and easy to implement. Consider the following as guidelines to help select and implement the right weight-loss diet:

Guideline #1: Every person on a weight-reduction diet should maintain a proper **nutrient** balance. For this reason, a diet that calls for the elimination of one or more categories of foods should be avoided. It is not the purpose of this book to explain how to balance a diet, but bear in mind that many good sources of information exist. Consult a family physician, talk to a registered dietician, or take college or university continuing-education courses.

Guideline #2: Selecting specific foods and creating a balanced

Nutrient: A nourishing component of food that serves to sustain life, promote growth, prevent decay, or provide energy.

overall diet are critical to any successful weight-loss plan. Two foods may be equally effective in providing a needed nutrient group to the diet, but there may be vast differences in their caloric value. For example, when selecting a food from the protein group, one could select roasted pork spareribs at 396 calories or the white meat of a roasted turkey for 132 calories. Both of these choices would provide the protein needed, but the turkey has 264 fewer calories.

Guideline #3: Preparation is another important element in choosing low-calorie foods. One half of a chicken breast, batter-fried with the skin on, contains about 360 calories, whereas the same chicken breast, roasted without the skin, contains only about 173 calories. In general, it is best to avoid foods that are fried, sautéed in butter, or served in cream sauce. Instead, include more foods that are baked, broiled, or steamed.

Guideline #4: The two real "no no's" on any weight reduction diet are foods high in **refined sugar** and high in fats. Some real diet disasters include deep-dish apple pie à la mode at 690 calories, pecan pie with whipped cream at 679 calories, or devil's food cake with fudge frosting for 409 calories. If a dessert is needed, try angel food cake with fresh strawberries for 163 calories. In addition, stay away from many cuts of meat, especially those with visible fat.

Guideline #5: To develop sound lifelong dietary practices and reduce body fat as well, include more vegetables, fruits, and complex carbohydrates in any eating pattern. **Complex carbohydrates** include such foods as whole grain cereals, breads, and pastas. In the past, certain fad diets tried to eliminate complex carbohydrates from weight-reduction programs, claiming that they were fat producers. In reality, carbohydrates contain 4 calories per gram, whereas fats contain 9 calories per gram. It has also been suggested that the calories derived from fats are more likely to turn into fat on the body than the calories derived from carbohydrates. Reducing fat intake and increasing complex carbohydrates in the diet is not just good advice for those trying to lose weight. According to U.S. Dietary Goals, many (if not most) Americans could benefit from this advice.

The "Fat Wheel" shown in figure 4.2 can be used to help make good food choices related to fats. Those foods listed near the center of the wheel are those lowest in fat and are the best choices. Each concentric ring out from the center indicates foods higher in fats. The wheel is also divided into groups of foods. Under each group name is a listing of the major nutrients found in that group.

Refined sugar: Term used to describe sweeteners such as white sugar that are created by processing and thus can be distinguished from natural sugars such as honey.

Complex carbohydrate: A polysaccharide, or compound consisting of many sugar molecules linked together. Complex carbohydrates in the diet include starches and the fiber, cellulose.

(continued on p. 70)

FIGURE 4.2
The Fat Wheel

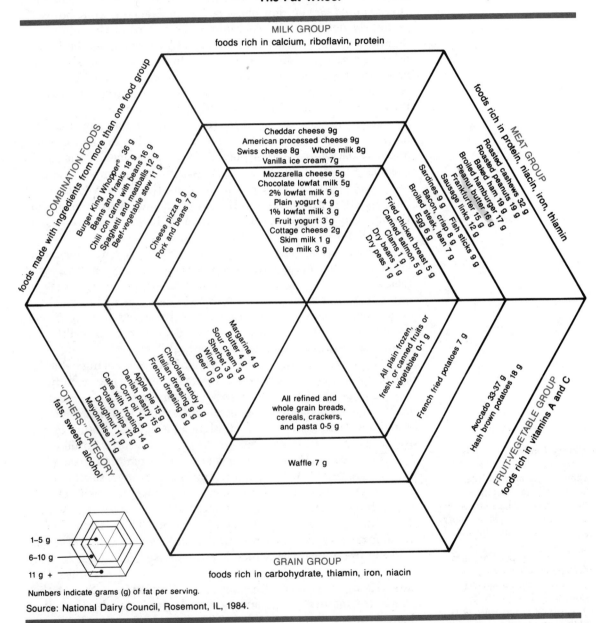

Numbers indicate grams (g) of fat per serving.

Source: National Dairy Council, Rosemont, IL, 1984.

The National Dairy Council's "fat wheel." Selecting a balanced set of foods from the center circle of the milk, meat, fruit-vegetable, and grain groups each day is a good way to obtain a low-fat diet.

BEYOND DIET

If losing excess fat were simply a matter of following a good diet, there should be very few obese people in America. This, however, is clearly not the case. As many as one-third of the adult U.S. population are overfat. To understand why, consider the host of other factors that come into play as soon as something as personal as eating behavior comes under discussion. People don't always consume food specifically because they are hungry or because they want to maintain an optimal state of health.

External cues can affect food selection, including such factors as the time of day, the smell of food, television advertisements, and food packaging and display. For example, consider the lure of the smell from a pizza house. Before smelling the pizza, you may not have been hungry, and while eating the pizza, you may not have been thinking about the calories you were consuming. Rather, the pizza's taste and smell may have been foremost in your mind.

Emotions such as guilt, boredom, loneliness, fear, depression, joy, and happiness may also influence the quantity and quality of food one selects. For example, a depressed person may crave a banana split or some other rich treat to help cheer him or her up. A joyous occasion can be celebrated by going out to dinner. Someone consuming foods on these occasions is probably not thinking about caloric input and output.

There are many other factors that influence eating behavior. For example, the eating habits a person has learned from his or her parents; the easy availability of many high-fat, high-calorie fast foods; the use of food for social gatherings; and the promotion and advertising on behalf of high-calorie snacks and **empty foods**, foods high in calories yet low in nutritional value.

The idea of food advertisement and promotion deserves a closer examination. How many times have advertisements on television promoted a carrot or a nice healthy squash? On the other hand, how often do commercials for candy, carbonated beverages, potato chips, and the like appear? There almost seems to be a reverse correlation between the health quality of a food and the frequency with which it is advertised. The least healthy foods appear to be promoted the most. If one assumes that advertising has some effect on food selection and agrees that there are more advertisements for the **junk foods**, then it is logical to conclude that advertising and food promotion cause people to eat foods that are less healthy and more fattening.

Those trying to lose weight cannot ignore the psychological

Empty foods: Foods that contain a high number of calories but provide little or no nutritional benefit; alcoholic beverages are often cited as an example of empty foods; see also junk food.

Junk food: A popular term used to describe food that contains a high number of calories but is low in nutritional value, especially highly processed snack foods containing large amounts of refined sugar.

FIGURE 4.3
Junk Food

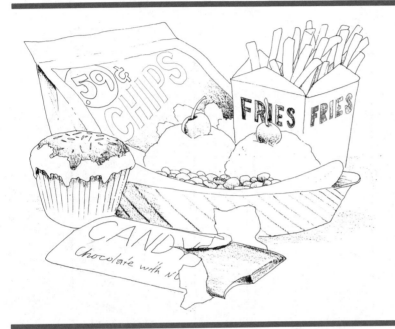

Millions of dollars are spent each year promoting high-fat, high-calorie, highly processed snacks and fast foods that have little or no nutritional value.

and behavioral factors associated with eating. Indeed, being aware of these factors—and learning to control them—is essential. This is not easy to do, however. Eating behavior is very personal, acquired over time, and deeply ingrained. The first step to take is to recognize the factors at work, then work to eliminate or control the ones identified to the best of one's ability. This process, called behavior modification, can help with the task of lifelong weight loss.

LIFELONG BEHAVIOR MODIFICATION

If the motivation to lose weight centers on fitting into a new swim suit by summer, body weight is always going to be a problem. As soon as that goal is met, previous eating habits will resurface and lost pounds will quickly be regained. Obviously, the ideal is to

(continued on p. 73)

FIGURE 4.4
Eating Behavior Chart

	FOOD	AMOUNT AND PREPARATION	TIME EATEN	ALONE SOCIAL (WITH WHOM?)	WHERE EATEN	MOOD A - Anxious B - Bored C - Tired D - Depressed E - Angry F - Good
BREAKFAST						
NOON						
EVENING						
EXTRAS						

Source: Alma Blake, "Group Approach to Weight Control: Behavior Modification, Nutrition, and Health Education," *Journal of the American Dietetic Association*, Vol. 69 (December 1976), p. 69.

The first step in a behavior modification weight-loss program is to determine one's daily caloric intake and eating patterns. This is often done by using a chart such as the one shown here to record food consumption for some specified period, usually a week or more.

reach the desired weight and maintain it. For this to occur, a lifelong change in eating and exercise patterns must take place. **Behavior modification** is an approach developed in the late 1960s to assist people in making such lifelong behavioral changes. It helps people recognize and understand their patterns of eating, then replaces unproductive patterns with new, improved behaviors conducive to lifelong weight control. [2]

The first step in behavior modification is to discern one's daily eating patterns. The chart in figure 4.4 is an example of the type of data needed. After filling in such a chart for a week or more, go back over it and identify undesirable behavior patterns. For example, a typical problem is snacking on high-calorie food while watching TV. This pattern could be replaced by snacking on low-calorie vegetables, doing needlework, or exercising while watching TV. Another problem might involve eating high-fat, high-calorie foods at fast-food restaurants when in a hurry. To counter this undesirable eating pattern, prepare in advance a variety of low-calorie foods that can be kept on hand in the refrigerator or freezer. Other undesirable patterns identified on the survey form should be changed in a similar manner.

Behavior modification techniques focus not only on eating, but on a whole range of behaviors closely related to eating as well. When buying food, it is important to use behavior modification techniques. Make a list of highly nutritious foods needed for a balanced diet and then shop only from the list. If foods high in calories are not readily available, they are easier to avoid. It has also been suggested that it may be helpful to shop after a meal because when one is full, those high-calorie snacks do not look nearly so tempting. Recent evidence, however, suggests there may be differences between the shopping behavior of the obese and their normal-weight counterparts. It seems the obese respond more to external stimuli than to their own internal signs of hunger. [3]

Behavior modification may also play a helpful role in the storage of food. Store foods in opaque containers and put them where they are difficult to get to. Remove all food from countertops and tables. Don't keep food in the living room or family room, where it is easily obtainable. Throw a small amount of food away rather than eating it simply because there is too little to save.

Behavior modification can be helpful when it comes to the preparation of food as well. Plan nutritious, low-calorie meals ahead of time. Avoid planning meals at the last minute, which often leads to selecting quick foods high in calories. Make only one serving of a food. If more food is desired after the first portion

Behavior modification: To alter one's behavior intentionally, eliminating unwanted behaviors, through a process of evaluating existing behaviors, identifying those to be changed, implementing changed behavior, and monitoring the results.

FIGURE 4.5
Appearances Do Matter

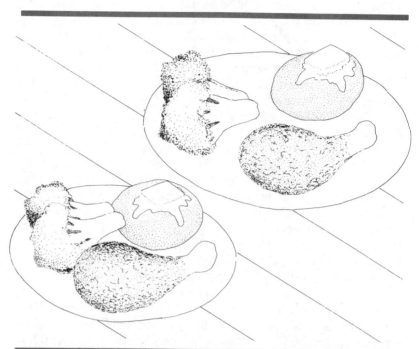

These two plates contain the same amounts of food. The smaller plate creates the illusion of more food and may help the dieter feel that he or she is eating more.

is eaten, another serving can always be made. However, the work of preparing more often will discourage you from having the extra serving. Avoid family-style servings and "all-you-can-eat" restaurants. They encourage overeating. Don't nibble while preparing food. A good nibbler can consume a significant number of calories before ever sitting down to eat.

Modify behavior when eating, too. Use smaller plates to make smaller servings look larger. Slow down the rate of eating. It takes 20 minutes for feelings of **satiety**, or fullness, to occur. To allow time for satiety, return eating utensils to the table between bites, chew food more thoroughly, and increase conversation at the table. These techniques help to slow eating behavior and will allow a sense of fullness to occur *before* a person consumes more than he or she needs.

Satiety: The feeling of fullness that follows eating.

(continued on p. 76)

Breaking the Chains that Lead to Overweight

We are creatures of habit. All of our behaviors are linked one to the next. Much like the chain that holds a boat to its anchor, our behavior chains can anchor us to relatively fixed conditions, like obesity. The chains can be simple or complicated, emotional or situation-specific.

An emotional chain might be formed by a stressful relationship, a disappointing date, an unpleasant conversation after a movie. Once the goodbyes are said, the distressed person, despite having dined out and had a couple of drinks, begins to snack.

And then there's the simple habit pattern. Consider the person who has, over the years, established a certain routine after shopping for food: he comes in the front door, carries the groceries to the kitchen, puts them in the cupboards and refrigerator—and then snacks. Soon, every time he comes in the front door and goes to the kitchen, he reaches for a snack.

Or consider the woman who comes home after a hard day at work. She puts down her briefcase, picks up the paper, turns on the TV, sits down, gets up and looks in the refrigerator, grabs a snack, sits back down in front of the TV, reads the paper and/or watches TV and snacks, and then eats a meal. After dinner, she sits down to watch TV, gets bored, walks into the kitchen, browses through the refrigerator, eats a piece of cheesecake.

All the specifics are different, but the patterns are similar. The behavior chain is a series of interconnected habitual behaviors. The beginning can be innocuous, such as a moment of stress or boredom, but the ending is always the same: extra calories.

How many eating situations in your life can you describe with a behavior chain diagram? A study of the series of linked events suggests a strategy for eliminating extra habitual eating or snacking. Break the chains. It's hard to just say no. The easy way to break the chain is to substitute an alternate activity. The earlier the chain is broken,

the better and the easier it will be to cut the calories. Once the snack touches your taste buds, it's too late. When that cheesecake is only a gleam in your eye or, even better, a pre-gleam, the awareness that you are headed for something to eat makes it easier to break the chain.

The way to cast off your chains is to identify them, pinpoint the weak links, and substitute another behavior. Using alternate activities sounds easy, but it's hard to do on the spur of the moment.

If your behavior chain is broken at any point, it will probably not continue. (The businesswoman's final behavior—eating, feeling guilty, eating—will probably not occur.) The earlier in the chain you substitute a nonfood link, the easier it is to intervene.

Four types of behavior can be substituted in an ongoing behavior chain:

1. Fun activities (grabbing your mate, taking a walk, reading a book).

2. Necessary activities (cleaning up a room, balancing your checkbook).

3. Incompatible activities (taking a shower).

4. Time-consuming activities (setting a kitchen timer for 20 minutes before allowing yourself to eat).

Using activities to interrupt behavior patterns that lead to inappropriate eating can be a powerful means of changing eating habits. This technique can also be useful when you are eating in response to environmental as well as internal cues for eating: for example, a TV ad for food or a hunger pang that you feel at an odd time after a meal or before going to bed. If it's pushing you to eat, substitute!

Several conditions have to be met before you succeed at chainbreaking. First, you have to identify the chain, pay attention to your habitual eating patterns, and see which patterns relentlessly recur in your daily life. Write down the behavior chain, starting with the eating or final behavior in the chain and work backwards to the beginning. The earliest behavior in the chain, for example, might be a boring TV show.

Second, you must have a list of alternative activities at hand. It's hard to remember what's fun, exciting, necessary, or even sexy when that piece of apple pie is warming up in the microwave. Have a list available of each kind of chain breaker so that you won't have to spend the time thinking about alternatives. Include at least three necessary, three pleasant, three incompatible, and three time-consuming alternatives on your list to use [when needed.]

Third, remember that hunger pangs triggered by your head rather than by your stomach are short-lived. (You'll gradually discern the crucial difference between the imagined, emotional need and the real, physical need to eat.) If you delay eating for 10 to 15 minutes, usually the urge to eat will diminish or disappear.

Finally, keep track of when you are successful. Pat yourself on the back for having counteracted the snacking reflex with some novel, noncaloric activity. With enough effort, snacking—which can add up to a colossal amount of calories—might not even be fun anymore.

—*James Ferguson, M.D.*

Source: *Healthline* (February 1990), pp. 2–3.

The principle of behavior modification applies to exercise as well. Analyze your current exercise patterns and alter these in helpful ways. Try exercising with a friend. The peer pressure can be very helpful. Plan exercise into the daily routine by picking a specific time to exercise and staying with it. If exercise is difficult during inclement weather, plan an alternative activity and be ready to use it. Using these and other similar strategies can help keep the exercise program going.

Self-Efficacy

Behavior modification can help a person develop lifelong behaviors necessary to reach and maintain his or her optimal weight, but other factors are also necessary. A 5-year follow-up of one weight-loss program revealed that the most successful weight-loss maintainers were those who adhered to behavioral procedures and were more physically active. [4] The most powerful predictor of positive weight status at post treatment and follow-up, however, appears to be **self-efficacy**, or a belief by the subjects that they have the ability to lose weight. Those who feel victimized by their weight, who believe it is out of their control, appear to lose less weight than those who are confident that they can lose weight. [5] Establishing self-efficacy may be one of the most important things a person can do to lose weight successfully.

Self-efficacy: A belief in one's ability to control events or to accomplish one's objectives; a sense of self-confidence.

MOTIVATION AND SKILLS TO SUCCEED

As a first step in reducing body fat, it is a good idea first to identify any current undesirable behaviors to establish a baseline against which to measure change. This can be accomplished by closely monitoring your current behavior. In the case of weight control, one should keep track of foods eaten and exercise patterns. Appropriate forms should be used to collect this data, and the self-monitoring should continue throughout the behavior change.

It is important that self-monitoring does not become so tedious or time-consuming that it discourages participation. Asking someone to keep track of everything they eat and to calculate the caloric and/or nutrient value of each food might be of value for a few days but not for the length of the program. Simply writing down foods eaten or recording exercise sessions is more realistic.

Although self-monitoring has been used primarily to assess current levels of behavior and to monitor change, there is evidence to indicate that it is also valuable in initiating change. The process of recording behavior increases one's awareness, which in and of itself can change behavior before any actual intervention has taken place. [6]

Setting Goals

Setting goals is an important part of any weight-loss program. [7] By doing this, individuals develop a concrete sense of what to strive for. Goals should be realistic and appropriate in order to be effective and motivating. Often those trying to lose weight underestimate the difficulty of a behavioral change and thus set unrealistic goals. For example, someone new to exercise may set a 3-mile daily run as a goal. Inappropriate goals such as this will usually lead to failure. Goals should be difficult enough to be challenging but not so difficult as to seem impossible. On the other hand, goals that are too easy to achieve may also be doomed to failure. [8]

A goal should state the specific **behavior** to be changed. It is important not to confuse behavior with outcomes at this juncture in the planning process. For example, it is not appropriate to have a goal of losing a certain number of pounds. This results from behavioral change, such as reducing dietary intake while increasing exercise. The behaviors a goal addresses should relate directly to diet and exercise and should be realistic. A person on a crash diet can successfully meet a weight-loss goal. But such a step is not a lifelong behavior change that will bring about a

Behavior: An observable action or response.

permanent alteration of body composition. Conversely, a person could follow the prescribed behavior change and not see a resulting weight loss. Behaviors that shift basal metabolism or enlarge the amount of muscle tissue could cause body weight to stabilize or even increase. [9]

For a goal to be effective it must be measurable and observable. In a weight-loss program, for example, a goal such as "I want to improve my health" should *not* be allowed. It is neither readily measurable nor observable. A much better goal would be "I will eat 1 additional vegetable and 1 additional fruit and eliminate all baked goods for the next 2 weeks." This behavior change can be observed and measured. Records can be kept to determine if the goal has been met. Stating specific behaviors does not change the anticipated outcome, that of improving the participant's health. It is up to the participant to decide whether or not the intervention is working. If the intervention is not effective, other behaviors should be altered to try to obtain the desired outcome. Most people need help establishing sound behavioral goals when first setting up a weight-loss program.

Goals should be set for various time frames. [10] For a person trying to reduce dietary fat, a short-range goal might be to avoid all fried foods for a day. An intermediate-range goal might be to eat only baked or broiled foods for a week or a month. A long-range goal, extending to 6 months or a year, may seek to eliminate all fried foods from the diet permanently. Short-range goals are particularly important as a person first tries to alter a behavior. It might be overwhelming to think of not eating french fries for 6 months, while the thought of not eating them for 24 hours might seem realistic. After a while the short-term goals may seem too easy and longer-range goals will be needed. Eventually the behavior should become such a normal part of the lifestyle that setting goals becomes unnecessary.

In general it is best not to try to change multiple behaviors at the same time. [11] It is tough enough to alter one behavior without trying to change several; therefore, someone trying to lose weight should not stop smoking at the same time. The one exception to this is when a second behavior change supports the first. For example, when the desired outcome is to lose weight, dietary intake behaviors complement exercise behaviors and both changes should be encouraged simultaneously.

Self-Rewards and Reinforcements

After one has set goals, it is a good idea to develop a set of reinforcements as a reward for meeting those goals. [12] For rewards to be effective, they must be valued, feasible, contingent upon predetermined rules, and immediate. [13] At the same time, the reward should not be too large. Some suggest that the behavior might then become too dependent on the external reward. If so, the participant may "rebound" to his or her original pattern of behavior when the reward is discontinued. [14]

For a reward system to be effective it must also be feasible. A trip to Europe might be highly valued, but if the individual devising the reward cannot afford such a trip, the reward will not work. Rewards using money are easy for most people to come up with, but unless the money is available they are not feasible.

Contingency is another important element of reward systems. The goal to be met to receive the reward must be clearly stated. If the goal is not met, the reward should not be granted. For example, if the goal is to exercise 5 out of 7 days a week for the next 6 weeks to obtain a new running suit, and the person only runs 5 of 7 days for 3 of the 6 weeks, the running suit should not be purchased. Certainly a new goal can be established with the same reward, but one should not be rewarded when he or she fails to meet a goal.

A reward should be received immediately after a goal has been met. [15] If one is going to buy a new compact disc for maintaining a well-balanced, 1,500-calorie diet for 7 days, he or she should not have to wait 2 weeks until payday to get the CD. Either the money to buy the CD should be set aside for such an event or another reward should be devised. Immediate reinforcement is an important element in the behavioral change process.

A final criterion for an effective reward system is that it must be used. One study of compliance rates among women who were asked to perform a breast self-examination found that women using self-rewards had rates of compliance similar to women receiving external rewards. Women who did not use self-rewards had compliance rates similar to the "no reinforcement" control group. [16] When people do not choose to provide themselves with self-reinforcements, it may be that such reinforcements are perceived as being trivial, unimportant, or as involving too much effort. These perceptions must be overcome if self-rewards are to be effective in reinforcing behavioral change.

Participants in weight-loss programs often need help developing good reward systems. Sadly, the first reward many such people think of is high-calorie, high-fat food. For example, people often think of going out for a big dinner or having a rich dessert as a reward for sticking to their diets. This is not only inappropriate but actually conflicts with the goal of the program. Money, or

Did You Know That . . .

Some obese people in a Stanford University study lost 2$\frac{1}{2}$ times as much weight as others. These more successful patients carried portable microcomputers to monitor their meals, snacks, and exercise, which provided them with immediate, continuous feedback.

rewards bought with money, may also serve as a reinforcement for success. That's fine as long as the reward meets the criteria of desirability, feasibility, contingency, and immediacy. If it doesn't, then nonmonetary reinforcers need to be explored.

Contracting

The process of **contracting** involves setting forth one's goals, rewards, and contingencies in a written document signed by one or more witnesses. [17] Contracting should be used for two distinct reasons. First, it forces people to formalize their goals and rewards. Second, it makes the behavioral change public. Now the behavioral-change goals are not just within the participant's mind because they have been stated in front of witnesses. It is much harder to break a contract with witnesses than it is to break a promise to oneself.

Selecting the proper witnesses is an important element in the contracting process. The witnesses must be people who know the participant well and can monitor his or her progress. It is not appropriate to ask other program participants to sign if they are only seen once a week during the class. It would be far better to have a spouse, parent, roommate, or close friend sign as a witness.

Force-Field Analysis

Before initiating a weight-loss program, it is important for participants to identify what forces or factors will help them to be successful in their behavioral change and what forces or factors will work against them. [18] An honest appraisal of these factors can help one to identify potential problem areas as well as potential areas of support. The idea is to minimize the effects of the negative factors and maximize the effects of the positive factors.

Consider a concrete example of this technique at work involving Phoebe, who has decided to initiate a walking program for physical fitness. Phoebe anticipates this should be an easy task during the summer and early fall but that walking outside in the cold weather is neither desirable nor likely. Phoebe may then start thinking of alternative options to use during the winter months. She can try another form of exercise—join a health club, for example, or buy a treadmill that could be used at home, or join a group of mall walkers. After weighing all the alternatives, Phoebe decides to join the group of walkers at the local shopping mall. This solution minimizes the negative factor of winter and has the potential to be a positive factor in that other walkers may

Contracting: The practice of drawing up an agreement (usually written) between two or more persons for the purpose of assigning responsibility for carrying out a particular task or activity and establishing the conditions under which this is to occur.

(continued on p. 82)

Behavior-Intervention Form

I State behavior to be changed/maintained

II Reasons for changing/maintaining this behavior
   1.
   2.
   3.

III Identify your current baseline for this behavior

IV State behavior change in the form of a precise behavioral goal (objective)

V Describe short-term rewards and contingencies

VI Describe intermediate and long-term rewards and contingencies

VII List positive forces that will help you change the behavior and negative forces that will hinder you:

   Positive   Negative

VIII Devise a record-keeping system appropriate for your intervention and attach it to this form

IX Complete the behavioral contract and attach it to this form

Did You Know That . . .

I f you team up with a partner to diet, you're likely to drop 30 percent more weight than someone who goes it alone, says a Purdue University study.

Behavioral Contract

I _____

Agree to: _____

_____

_____

_____

_____

For the period from _____ to _____

If I perform the behavior I will reward myself as follows:

_____

_____

_____

_____

_____

If I do not perform the above behavior, I agree to forgo the above reward.

Signed: _____ Date: _____
Witness # 1: _____ Date: _____
Witness # 2: _____ Date: _____
Witness # 3: _____ Date: _____

provide social support to continue with the program. The point is that instead of waiting until it was too cold to walk and then discontinuing the program, Phoebe has identified a potential problem early and has solved it in a very positive way.

Behavioral-Intervention Forms
One way to incorporate a variety of strategies into a behavioral-change program is through the use of a behavioral-intervention form. The purpose of completing such a form is to structure the behavioral-change process so it will include multiple strategies to help maximize a person's chances of obtaining his or her goals. A sample of such a form appears on the top of page 81.

On line 1, subjects are asked to state the behavior they would like to change. At this point it is important to be sure participants are really trying to change a behavior and not obtain an outcome. Looking more fit is not a behavior; increasing exercise is. Feeling more relaxed is not a behavior; practicing neuromuscular-relaxation training is.

Next, the participant is asked to list 3 reasons for changing the behavior. These reasons can be used to reinforce the behavioral change as time goes on. If the person starts to falter, the reasons can be reexamined to determine if they have changed or if they are still strong enough to motivate continued participation. The reasons stated can also be a clue to the likelihood of success in the program. A participant once listed his 3 reasons for trying to lose weight as "my parents wanted me to lose weight," "my wife wants me to lose weight," and "my doctor wants me to lose weight." When asked if he wanted to lose weight, his reply was "No, I really enjoy eating and cooking." As might be expected, he was not successful in his attempt to lose weight. The reasons why he was attempting to lose weight were not his own. In another case, the main reason a college woman wanted to lose weight was to fit into her swimsuit. At one point during her program, she was overheard telling a friend, "I cannot wait to reach my desired weight so I can eat what I want again."

Obviously, her reason for losing weight, although strong enough to provide initial success, was not going to produce a permanent life-style change.

Self-monitoring is included in step III, when the participant is asked to identify a baseline of the current behavior. Next, some type of record-keeping system should be set up to follow and evaluate this behavior for approximately one week. Using this information, goals will be set. The same record-keeping system may be used, if appropriate, in step VIII.

In step IV, a goal is set. This is a critical step. Considerable time should be taken to ensure that goals are realistic and feasible. Once appropriate goals are set, self-rewards and reinforcers can be established in steps V and VI.

A force-field analysis is conducted in step VII. The positive forces identified should be used to reinforce the behavioral change. Meanwhile, steps should be taken to minimize the impact of the negative forces identified.

Finally, the participant is required to complete a behavioral-change contract. A sample behavioral-change contract is provided on page 81.

Mind-Set

When beginning a diet or a behavior-modification program, **mind-set** is extremely important. Mind-set refers to a preconceived expectation regarding weight loss when entering a program. These expectations can become so rigid that they actually set one up for failure.

Reaching the desired weight is going to take time. Periods when weight loss is slower or a plateau is reached where no weight loss will occur for a time are common. If the mind-set is that weight loss should continue as long as one adheres to the diet, one can expect to be frustrated and tempted to abandon the program.

Another mind-set problem centers on the notion that the dieter must behave perfectly, eating only the right foods for the rest of his or her life. Although it is true that the behavioral changes made in a program are to be lifelong, it does not mean dieters can never taste their favorite foods again. Certainly they cannot have them as often, or perhaps in portions as large as before. But an occasional dessert or large meal does not spell failure. If an occasion for overeating arises, such as a holiday, compensate by eating less before and after the occasion. Even those who really go overboard and overeat in the extreme can adopt a mind-set of relapse, not of failure.

(continued on p. 86)

Did You Know That . . .

A Duke University psychologist found that food flavor is important to most people, but may be even more crucial to the overweight, who need many different tastes to feel satisfied. She adds a calorie-free flavor enhancer to bland food for dieters.

Mind-set: An established attitude or inclination toward a subject or situation.

Many "losers" know the pattern all too well. After the first several weeks of shedding pounds, they reach a point below which their weight will not budge—despite their following a strict dietary regimen to the calorie—and they give up in despair. What these dieters don't realize is that if the needle on the scale gets "stuck," it doesn't necessarily mean they are incapable of losing more weight. It may

When a Dieter Hits a Stubborn Plateau

simply have to do with the fact that the more a dieter reduces, the fewer calories he or she must consume (or the more that must be burned through exercise) in order to keep on losing; the original calorie limit may no longer suffice.

The reason is that bigger, or heavier, bodies need more calories than smaller ones to carry around the extra weight, according to William Rumpler, PhD, a physiologist who recently measured the calorie-burning rates of a group of obese men at the U.S. Department of Agriculture's Human Nutrition Research Center in Beltsville, Maryland. Consider, for example, a 200-pound man who easily loses 20 pounds, or 10 percent of his body weight, on a 2,500-calorie diet.

Once he's down to 180 pounds, his newly trimmed body will need about 10 percent fewer calories to maintain itself than it did when it tipped the scale at 200. That's because when healthy people lose 10 percent of their poundage they require about 10 percent fewer calories in order to remain at their new weight. Thus, if the man wants to keep on losing weight at the same rate until he reaches, say, 160, he will have to cut the calorie intake on his weight loss regimen by an additional 10 percent for a daily limit of 2,250 calories—or burn an extra 250 calories through an increase in exercise. What it boils down to is that "if you start out at 200 pounds and want to weigh 160, you have to eat like a 160-pounder, not a 180-pounder," Dr. Rumpler says.

There are other variables, to be sure. Some researchers believe, for instance, that much of the reason dieters hit plateaus is that the body resists weight loss, which it perceives as "starvation," by lowering its metabolism—that is, the rate at which it burns calories to breathe, digest food, and perform the other work that keeps it functioning. Still, before surrendering efforts to lose more weight to a "slowed" metabolism, a successful "early loser" should assess whether the number of calories he eats—and burns—on his diet and exercise plan has changed any since he first obtained a svelter physique and make adjustments from there so that he can be an even better "loser" in the long run.

Source: *Tufts University Diet & Nutrition Letter,* Vol. 8, No. 3, May 1990, p. 1.

FIGURE 4.6
Four Diets: How They Compare After One Year

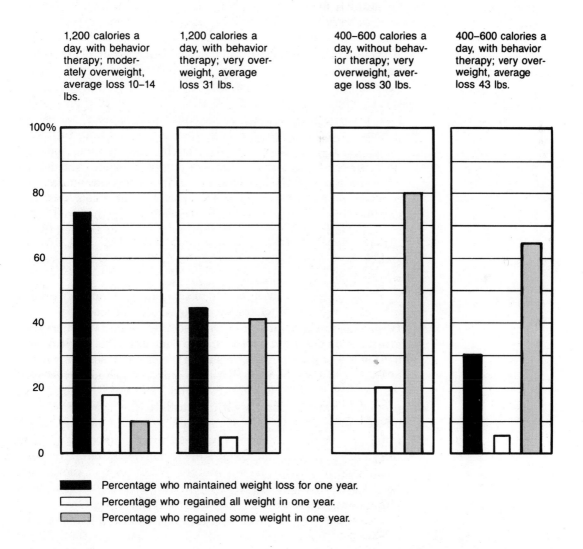

1,200 calories a day, with behavior therapy; moderately overweight, average loss 10–14 lbs.

1,200 calories a day, with behavior therapy; very overweight, average loss 31 lbs.

400–600 calories a day, without behavior therapy; very overweight, average loss 30 lbs.

400–600 calories a day, with behavior therapy; very overweight, average loss 43 lbs.

■ Percentage who maintained weight loss for one year.
☐ Percentage who regained all weight in one year.
▨ Percentage who regained some weight in one year.

Source: Deborah Blumenthal, "Dieting Reassessed," *New York Times Magazine* (9 October 1988), p. 24.

As demonstrated by the results from a recent study portrayed above, the diets that work best over the long run (in this case one year) tend to combine a gradual approach to weight loss with behavior modification therapy.

The difference between relapse and failure is important. After a bad day, when the diet is blown, the relapse mind-set requires one to think about getting back on the proper diet tomorrow. On the other hand, if a mind-set of failure prevails, thoughts will be of doom and despair and previous eating patterns might well be resumed.

Diet-Help Industry

Although the basic concepts of diet and weight control are easy to understand, sticking to them is a difficult matter for many overweight people. As a result, a large array of products and services have been developed to assist people with their weight-loss programs. These products and services can be loosely grouped together into what is known as the **diet-help industry**. Many products and services offered by the diet-help industry have proven track records and are helpful to some, but not all, who use them. It is important to remember that *no diet-help program or product can guarantee success*. The major factor in determining success is still the person using the product or service. Hard work and determination are needed to stick to any program. If the person using the product or service loses motivation or does not follow program guidelines, the diet-help program will fail for him or her.

The largest and best known of the diet-help industry organizations is Weight Watchers, owned by the giant food corporation H. J. Heinz. Dieticians have praised the Weight Watchers' program for its balanced approach, one that promotes healthy diet, behavior modification, group support, and exercise. Competitors of Weight Watchers in the diet-help industry include Overeaters Anonymous, TOPS, Nutri/System, and Diet Center. Each of these programs varies greatly with regard to the type of services offered and cost. As a rule, if one can lose weight on one's own, it is best to do so. For those who need group support and basic information, TOPS and Overeaters Anonymous offer the least expensive quality programs. Weight Watchers is a moderately priced program, while Nutri/System and Diet Center tend to be more structured and more expensive. [10] (See page 87.)

The diet-help industry is a big business. Estimates of total revenues range upward from $3 billion a year. In 1988, Weight Watchers had revenues of $1.3 billion, and its $100 million operating income represented 14.5 percent of parent company Heinz's income. Weight Watchers is so big and so successful that Heinz has called it "our growth engine for the 1990s." [20] Revenues for Weight Watchers come not only from the programs,

(continued on p. 89)

Diet-help industry: The industry comprised of those firms and other organizations that produce and market programs, diet aids, and other materials or services designed to promote weight loss.

A Guide to the Nationwide Programs

We asked several weight-loss experts to comment on the nationally based weight-loss programs. One conclusion: The best programs also tend to be the least expensive. However, the experts are careful to point out that motivation for losing weight takes different forms. You may find that one of the more-expensive, more-structured programs provides the spur you need to take weight off and keep it off.

Among the popular programs, TOPS and Overeaters Anonymous are informal, low-cost, nonprofit groups. Weight Watchers is moderate in cost and amount of structure. Nutri-System and Diet Center are more expensive and their diets are highly restrictive. The strictest—and most expensive—are liquid diets, such as Optifast. You should consider them only if you're at least 40 pounds to 50 pounds overweight and have tried food-based programs without success.

The big-name programs have a professional staff at headquarters, but their local groups are usually run by graduates of the program, who have little or no professional training.

TOPS (Take Off Pounds Sensibly)
414-482-4620
P.O. Box 07360
Milwaukee, Wis. 53207
MEETINGS: weekly group meetings
APPROXIMATE COST: weekly, 25 cents to 50 cents a week; yearly, $12; after two years, $10 per year
SPECIAL FOODS: none; you follow recommendations from your physician

Camaraderie, competition and recognition help motivate members of TOPS, a loosely structured network of local groups with nearly 12,000 chapters in the U.S. and other countries. Weekly meetings consist of a weigh-in, followed by an upbeat program that stresses motivation and positive reinforcement. Unpaid volunteers direct the meetings. Each chapter has a different approach and should be evaluated individually.

Members must see their own physicians to set weight-loss goals and a dietary regimen.

"Before" and "after" photos of TOPS weight-loss contest winners appear annually in the club's national magazine, which also prints news tips and simple recipes.

About 13% of members manage to maintain their weight goal for 13 weeks, which makes them members of KOPS (Keep Off Pounds Sensibly).

OVEREATERS ANONYMOUS
213-542-8363
P.O. Box 92870
Los Angeles, Cal. 90009
MEETINGS: weekly group meetings
APPROXIMATE COST: none
SPECIAL FOODS: none

The focus of OA is not on weight, calories or dieting but on learning to stop eating compulsively. Members follow a 12-step plan patterned after that of Alcoholics Anonymous, which focuses on their emotional and spiritual life. There are no rules, but members are encouraged to see a physician for medical and dietary guidance. An OA survey found that 78% of members lose at least ten pounds, with an average loss of 50 pounds. About 10% of those members have maintained their weight loss for five years. Most OA members are 50 pounds to 100 pounds overweight when they join. They're usually feeling desperate, says Carol Hilliard, OA's publications and communications manager. Many have tried other diets and weight-loss programs without lasting success. OA can be a great source of emotional support, says Evelyn Tribole, a registered dietitian and representative of the American Dietetic Association. She recommends it to clients who need a low-cost alternative to counseling. Members are encouraged to call each other, and it's not unusual for everyone to join hands at the end of a meeting and say a prayer. Chapters differ in their emotional tone, so Tribole recommends trying different groups to find one you can identify with.

NUTRI/SYSTEM

215-784-7900
3901 Commerce Ave.
Willow Grove, Pa. 19090
MEETINGS: weekly, meet individually with a nutritionist; group meeting with a behaviorist
APPROXIMATE COST: $300 to $400 to lose 30 to 40 pounds, plus about $50 per week for food
SPECIAL FOODS: prepackaged foods and flavor powders sold by the company; vitamin supplements

The company supplies your meals each week in proportioned packages. Many of the entrees— and the desserts—are flavored with NutraSweet.

The program is based on a theory that overweight people feel deprived of flavor, so they overeat. "It's very expensive, but it's the easiest way I've ever lost weight," says Robin Levey, a New York graduate of the program who went from 140 pounds to 125. Because she lives alone and hates to cook, Levey liked the convenience of prepackaged food. But it reduced her flavor cravings in an odd way. "Some of it tasted so bad, it taught me not to feel I have to finish everything on my plate," she says. Once you reach your desired weight, weekly visits taper off to once a month during the one-year maintenance program. If you gain back no more than five pounds in a year, you get back 50% of the program fee. The company claims that nearly everyone who keeps coming for a year keeps the weight off, but won't divulge the drop-out rate.

WEIGHT WATCHERS

Check your local phone listing
500 North Broadway
Jericho, N.Y. 11753
MEETINGS: weekly group meetings
APPROXIMATE COST: registration, $12 to $20; weekly meeting, $8
SPECIAL FOODS: none

Nutrition specialists count Weight Watchers among the best programs because the good habits you acquire while losing weight can also help you keep the pounds off. Its flexible food plan uses ordinary store-bought foods, which you must weigh according to Weight Watchers guidelines. The plan includes drinking at least eight glasses of water a day. Weight Watcher-brand foods are available but not required. They are, however, implicitly endorsed through discount coupons distributed at meetings. H. J. Heinz, which owns Weight Watchers International, has no specific dietary guidelines for products with the Weight Watchers' label, and many of the desserts contain a high amount of saturated fat.

Dietitians tout the fact that Weight Watchers lets you run your own program. Each day, you keep track of your meals in a booklet that sets out what you're allowed from each food group. Your choices and calorie intake expand each week for the first five weeks. You're also allowed "optional calories." You could lose as much as ten pounds in the first week, but the rate should taper off to less than two pounds per week.

The exercise plan is optional. Like the food plan, it presents choices and provides suggestions but leaves the initiative up to you.

DIET CENTER

208-356-9381
220 South Second West
Rexburg, Idaho 83440
MEETINGS: individual counseling daily for first several weeks, then weekly; weekly group meetings
APPROXIMATE COST: $400 to $650 to lose 25 pounds; $600 to $950 to lose 36 pounds
SPECIAL FOODS: protein food supplements

Private counseling six days a week is central to this highly structured approach. The plan eliminates dairy products and adds a food supplement of soy protein, sugar and B-complex vitamins. You'll also be offered other Diet Center vitamins and food products; They're a major source of profit.

Upon reaching your weight goal, you stop taking the food supplement and begin a "stabilization" period of up to three weeks that includes counseling every two days and gradual reintroduction of normal foods. You continue seeing your counselor at weekly sessions for a year.

Throughout the program, you keep an exercise diary and attend weekly group sessions to view videotaped lessons on meal planning, stress management and exercise.

Some dietitians, including Tribole, question the balance of Diet Center's eating plan. "Eliminating dairy products is unnecessary and doesn't promote normal eating," says Tribole, who also argues that the diet's emphasis on protein, and especially meat, makes it harder to maintain weight loss.

OPTIFAST
800-328-5392
5320 W. 23rd St. P.O. Box 370
Minneapolis, Minn. 55440
MEETINGS: weekly discussion group; weekly checkup with physician
APPROXIMATE COST: $2,500 to $3,000 for six months
SPECIAL FOODS: liquid meals

Optifast is a very low-calorie liquid diet for moderate to severe obesity. You must be at least 30% or 50 pounds overweight to sign up. Medical and psychological evaluations are required because severe obesity is usually accompanied by medical problems, such as diabetes or hypertension.

You get powdered meals to mix with water—420 calories a day. After 12 weeks, you begin adding fish and poultry. Aerobic exercise is encouraged, and the supplements are phased out as you approach goal weight. About 60% to 70% of participants complete the six-month program, according to Sandoz Nutrition, which makes the meals.

Participants are examined regularly by a physician and attend classes run by a behavioral psychologist and a registered dietitian. For an additional $500, you can continue to attend group meetings and have your diet and exercise monitored for six months after you reach goal weight.

Like all liquid diets, Optifast, while rigorous and expensive, may be ineffective in the long term. Nutritionists caution against trying any liquid diet unless the plan is administered under close medical supervision and includes an exercise program and behavioral counseling.

Source: *Changing Times,* April 1989, pp. 79–80.

but also from the Weight Watchers brand of food that sold $780 million in 1988. One advantage to Weight Watchers is that participants do not have to purchase Weight Watchers foods to be in the program. Competitors such as Nutri/System and Jenny Craig centers require participants to purchase their brands of foods. Although it is convenient for people to have prepackaged prepared meals, it adds to the cost of the program, as foods average from $50 to $65 per week. In addition, by using these prepackaged diet foods, the participant is not learning how to develop the lifelong dietary habits needed to maintain his or her desired weight.

Concerns have also been raised about the safety of programs using these prepackaged diet foods. Counselors for the programs are usually not trained health-care professionals. They often advocate unsafe dietary practices. Before joining any program, one should check with a family physician or dietician for advice on the program being considered.

(continued on p. 94)

The Diet Readiness Test

To see how well your attitudes equip you for a weight-loss program, answer the questions below and on the following pages. For each question, circle the answer that best describes your attitude. As you complete each of the six sections, tally your score and analyze it according to the scoring guide below it.

I. Goals, Attitudes and Readiness

1. Compared to previous attempts, how motivated to lose weight are you this time?

1	2	3	4	5
Not at all motivated	Slightly motivated	Somewhat motivated	Quite motivated	Extremely motivated

2. How certain are you that you will *stay* committed to a weight-loss program for the time it will take to reach your goal?

1	2	3	4	5
Not at all certain	Slightly certain	Somewhat certain	Quite certain	Extremely certain

3. Considering all outside factors at this time in your life—the stress you're feeling at work, your family obligations, etc.—to what extent can you tolerate the effort required to stick to a diet?

1	2	3	4	5
Cannot tolerate	Can tolerate somewhat	Uncertain	Can tolerate well	Can tolerate easily

4. Think honestly about how much weight you hope to lose and how quickly you hope to lose it. Figuring a weight loss of 1 to 2 pounds per week, how realistic is your expectation?

1	2	3	4	5
Very unrealistic	Somewhat unrealistic	Moderately unrealistic	Somewhat realistic	Very realistic

5. While dieting, do you fantasize about eating a lot of your favorite foods?

1	2	3	4	5
Always	Frequently	Occa-sionally	Rarely	Never

6. While dieting, do you feel deprived, angry and/or upset?

1	2	3	4	5
Always	Frequently	Occa-sionally	Rarely	Never

If you scored:

6 to 16: This may not be a good time for you to start a diet. Inadequate motivation and commitment and unrealistic goals could block your progress. Think about what contributes to your unreadiness and consider changing these factors before undertaking a diet.

17 to 23: You may be close to being ready to begin a program but should think about ways to boost your preparedness.

24 to 30: The path is clear: You can decide *how* to lose weight in a safe, effective way.

Note: This test is designed to provide you with a rough idea of whether it is a good time for you to begin a diet. It was developed from the author's experience with hundreds of dieters at his clinic at the University of Pennsylvania and from the findings of other researchers. But neither this nor any other currently available test should be used as the only basis for your decision. Rather it should be viewed as a tool to help you ask yourself the right questions. In the end, however, you will be the best judge of your readiness to diet.

II. Hunger and Eating Cues

7. When food comes up in conversation or in something you read, do you want to eat even if you are not hungry?

1	2	3	4	5
Never	Rarely	Occa-sionally	Frequently	Always

8. How often do you eat because of *physical hunger*?

1	2	3	4	5
Always	Frequently	Occa-sionally	Rarely	Never

9. Do you have trouble controlling your eating when your favorite foods are around the house?

1	2	3	4	5
Never	Rarely	Occa-sionally	Frequently	Always

If you scored:

3 to 6: You might occasionally eat more than you'd like, but it does not appear to be due to high responsiveness to environmental cues. Controlling the attitudes that make you eat may be especially helpful.

7 to 9: You may have a moderate tendency to eat just because food is available. Dieting may be easier for you if you try to resist external cues and eat only when you are physically hungry.

10 to 15: Some or much of your eating may be in response to thinking about food or exposing yourself to temptations to eat. Think of ways to minimize your exposure to temptation so you eat only in response to physical hunger.

III. Control over Eating

If the following situations occurred while you were on a diet, would you be likely to eat *more* or *less* immediately afterward and for the rest of the day?

10. Although you planned on skipping lunch, a friend talks you into going out for a midday meal.

1	2	3	4	5
Would eat much less	Would eat somewhat less	Would make no differ-ence	Would eat somewhat more	Would eat much more

11. You "break" your diet by eating a fattening, "forbidden" food.

1	2	3	4	5
Would eat much less	Would eat somewhat less	Would make no differ-ence	Would eat somewhat more	Would eat much more

12. You have been following your diet faithfully and decide to test yourself by eating something you consider a treat.

1	2	3	4	5
Would eat much less	Would eat somewhat less	Would make no differ-ence	Would eat somewhat more	Would eat much more

If you scored:

3 to 7:   You recover rapidly from mistakes. However, if you frequently alternate between eating out of control and dieting very strictly, you may have a serious eating problem and should get professional help.

8 to 11:   You do not seem to let unplanned eating disrupt your program. This is a flexible, balanced approach.

12 to 15:   You may be prone to overeat after an event breaks your control or throws you off the track. Your *reaction* to these problem-causing eating events can be improved.

IV. Binge Eating and Purging

13. Aside from holiday feasts, have you ever eaten a large amount of food rapidly and felt afterward that this eating incident was excessive and out of control?

2	0
Yes	No

14. If yes to #13, how often have you engaged in this behavior during the last year?

1	2	3	4	5	6
Less than once a month	About once a month	A few times a month	About once a week	About three times a week	Daily

15. Have you ever purged (used laxatives, diuretics or induced vomiting) to control your weight?

5	0
Yes	No

16. If yes to #15, how often have you engaged in this behavior during the last year?

1	2	3	4	5	6
Less than once a month	About once a month	A few times a month	About once a week	About three times a week	Daily

If you scored:

0:   It appears that binge eating and purging is not a problem for you.

2 to 11:   Pay attention to these eating patterns. Should they arise more frequently, get professional help.

12 to 19:   You show signs of having a potentially serious eating problem. See a counselor experienced in evaluating eating disorders right away.

V. Emotional Eating

17. Do you eat more than you would like to when you have negative feelings such as anxiety, depression, anger or loneliness?

1	2	3	4	5
Never	Rarely	Occasionally	Frequently	Always

18. Do you have trouble controlling your eating when you have positive feelings—do you celebrate feeling good by eating?

1	2	3	4	5
Never	Rarely	Occasionally	Frequently	Always

19. When you have unpleasant interactions with others in your life, or after a difficult day at work, do you eat more than you'd like?

1	2	3	4	5
Never	Rarely	Occa-sionally	Frequently	Always

If you scored:

3 to 8:   You do not appear to let emotions affect your eating.

9 to 11:   You sometimes eat in response to emotional highs and lows. Monitor this behavior to learn when and why it occurs and be prepared to find alternate activities.

12 to 15:   Emotional ups and downs can stimulate your eating. Try to deal with the feelings that trigger the eating and find other ways to express them.

VI. Exercise Patterns and Attitudes

20. How often do you exercise?

1	2	3	4	5
Never	Rarely	Occa-sionally	Somewhat	Frequently

21. How confident are you that you can exercise regularly?

1	2	3	4	5
Not at all confident	Slightly confident	Somewhat confident	Highly confident	Completely confident

22. When you think about exercise, do you develop a positive or negative picture in your mind?

1	2	3	4	5
Completely negative	Somewhat negative	Neutral	Somewhat positive	Completely positive

23. How certain are you that you can work regular exercise into your daily schedule?

1	2	3	4	5
Not at all certain	Slightly certain	Somewhat certain	Quite certain	Extremely certain

If you scored:

4 to 10:   You're probably not exercising as regularly as you should. Determine whether your attitude about exercise or your lifestyle is blocking your way, then change what you must and put on those walking shoes!

11 to 16:   You need to feel more positive about exercise so you can do it more often. Think of ways to be more active that are fun and fit your lifestyle.

17 to 20:   It looks like the path is clear for you to be active. Now think of ways to get motivated.

After scoring yourself in each section of this questionnaire you should be able to better judge your dieting strengths and weaknesses. Remember that the first step in changing eating behavior is to understand the conditions that influence your eating habits.

Source: K. D. Brownell, *The Weight Control Digest*, Vol. 1, 1990, pp. 6–8.

The behavior-modification technique of chewing slowly to lose weight started at the turn of the century with Horace Fletcher, the "Great Masticator." He advised chewing every mouthful of food to a liquid pulp, to keep the colon clean.

In addition to these major programs, there are a host of smaller ones. All of these smaller programs should be evaluated carefully. A lucrative market such as the diet-help industry is bound to attract its share of quacks, charlatans, and hucksters. Many small local programs provide valuable assistance to those seeking weight loss, but others are provided only to make money for their founders and promote questionable, even fraudulent, practices.

Adherence Strategies

One major problem with individual weight-loss programs is that people often lose their motivation, give up, and drop out. This happens much less often in group programs that require cash deposits for attendance. [21] Many of the programs return the entire deposit or a portion of the deposit to the client based on attendance. A related strategy is to make the refunds contingent on group performance (that is, weight loss) rather than on individual weight loss or attendance. It has been found that group contracts are associated with significantly more weight loss than individual contracts, and this difference was maintained over a 1-year follow-up. No doubt social support and peer influences play a role in this finding. It appears that small deposits, from $30 to $300, produce poor short-term treatment outcomes. Larger deposits produce better initial results. The short-term advantage of the larger contracts, however, disappeared rapidly with time. [22]

Diet and behavior modification are two critical elements of a weight-control program. In developing a good diet, it is important to include a variety of foods in order to create a healthy, nutritionally balanced eating plan. Calories are important to weight loss. As a result, foods should be selected that have high nutrient values with low-calorie content. In general, foods high in fats and refined sugars should be avoided.

Behavior-modification techniques help identify and overcome poor eating patterns that have become part of life. They help establish new eating patterns, ones more conducive to proper weight control. Dieters can use behavior-modification techniques when purchasing, preparing, eating, and storing food. Such techniques can also help maintain an exercise program.

If a person has difficulty maintaining a diet, the diet-help industry can provide a host of products and services. Group support, provided through various organizations and programs, can be quite valuable in helping one stick to a diet. Diet-help programs can also assist in developing a proper mind-set for lifelong, permanent weight loss. ⬛

Fads, Gimmicks, Gadgets, and Quick Weight-Loss Programs

ONE NEED LOOK NO FURTHER than the headlines of the tabloids and magazines at the checkout counter of the local grocery store to get an idea of the number and quality of diets available. Most of these diets can legitimately be labeled **fad diets**.

FAD DIETS

Webster defines a fad as "a practice of interest followed for a time with exaggerated zeal." [1] This definition appropriately describes many diets. Fad diets are ones that attract the interest of overweight people who follow the diet's recommendations, usually for a short period of time, with great enthusiasm or zeal. People on a fad diet are usually quick to extol the virtues of the program to others, thus making the program very popular very quickly. For a time, it seems that everyone is on the particular diet. Then, a short while later, the diet is out of vogue and a new fad diet takes its place.

Literally millions of Americans attempt to lose weight using fad diets each year. The common attraction of most such diets is that they make losing weight seem simple and effortless. In addition, fad diet promoters frequently guarantee results and use well-known or well-toned personalities to endorse their diets. If indeed these diets worked as advertised, it would be a simple matter for the 80 million overfat Americans to lose weight. Unfortunately, this is not the case. Perhaps the most compelling

Fad diets: Weight-loss eating programs taken up and followed with exaggerated zeal for a short time.

(continued on p. 97)

95

Some Popular Weight-Loss Methods

Type of Method	Principle	Advantages	Disadvantages	Comments
Surgical procedures	Alteration of the gastrointestinal tract changes capacity or amount of absorptive surface	Caloric restriction is less necessary	Risks of surgery and postsurgical complications include death	Radical procedures include stapling of the stomach and removal of a section of the small intestine
Fasting	No energy input ensures negative energy balance	Weight loss is rapid (which may be a disadvantage) Exposure to temptation is reduced	**Ketogenic** A large portion of weight lost is from lean body mass Nutrients are lacking	Medical supervision is mandatory and hospitalization is recommended
Protein-sparing modified fast	Same as fasting except protein intake helps preserve lean body mass	Same as above	Ketogenic Nutrients are lacking Some unconfirmed deaths have been reported, possibly from potassium depletion	Medical supervision is mandatory Popular presentation was made in Linn's *The Last Chance Diet*
One-food-centered diets	Low caloric intake favors negative energy balance	Being easy to follow has initial psychological appeal	Nutrients are probably lacking Repetitious nature may cause boredom	No food or food combination is known to "burn off" fat Examples include the grapefruit diet and the egg diet
Low-carbohydrate, high-fat diets	Increased ketone excretion removes energy-containing substances from the body Fat intake is often voluntarily decreased; a low-calorie diet results	Inclusion of rich foods may have psychological appeal Initial rapid loss of water may be an incentive	Ketogenic High-fat intake is contraindicated for heart and diabetes patients Nutrients are often lacking	Popular versions have been offered by Taller and Atkins; some have been called the "Mayo," "Drinking Man's," and "Air Force" diets

Type of Method	Principle	Advantages	Disadvantages	Comments
Low-carbohydrate, high-protein diets	Low caloric intake favors negative energy balance		Expense and repetitious nature may make it difficult to sustain	If meat is emphasized, this diet is high in fat The Pennington diet is an example
High-carbohy-drate, low-fat diets	Low caloric intake favors negative energy balance	Wise food selections can make the diet nutritionally sound	Initial water retention may be discouraging	

Source: Patsy Bostick Reed, *Nutrition: An Applied Science* (St Paul: West Publishing, 1980).

evidence against fad diets is that so many new ones are developed constantly. It should be painfully obvious that if a truly simple and effortless method to lose weight were ever developed, everyone would take advantage of it and there would be no need for all the "new" diets.

Since rapid weight loss is one of the main motivating factors for using fad diets, it is important to examine this concept more closely. Rapid weight loss is generally considered to be unhealthy and unlikely to produce the desired long-term effects. By fasting or near fasting, a person can lose weight quickly, but a large portion of the weight is from lean body tissue and body fluids, not fat stores. In addition, fasting for more than a day or two can deplete the body of nutrients it needs on a daily basis. In other words, rapid weight loss can be harmful to one's health. It can even be fatal.

Fad-diet promoters use many different diets and diet ploys. The box above lists some of the more popular weight-loss methods, the principles under which they operate, and the advantages and disadvantages of each approach.

With all the fad diets available on the market, it is difficult to determine which are safe to use and which are not. Whenever in doubt, the first person to check with is a physician or a dietician. Do not be fooled by diets claiming to have the approval of the American Medical Association or a specific physician. This ploy is often used to get people to try fad diets. A doctor or a qualified dietician should be the judge. Next look at the foods allowed by the diet. Are choices from all 4 food groups included to

Ketogenic: Any behavior or activity that can cause ketosis, a potentially serious condition characterized by the accumulation of excessive amounts of ketone in the body. The symptoms of ketosis include irritability, weakness, and nausea.

Weight-Reduction Diet Evaluation Guide

Directions: Answer "yes" or "no" to each of the following questions:

_____ Does *your* M.D. or dietician approve of the weight-loss plan?

_____ Does the diet include the minimum number of servings from *each* of the 4 food groups?

_____ Does the diet include caloric restrictions?

_____ Does the diet include a good variety of foods to choose from?

_____ Are the foods inexpensive and easy to obtain?

_____ Does the diet limit weight loss to approximately 2 pounds per week?

_____ Does the weight-loss plan include lifelong behavior-modification techniques?

_____ Does the weight-loss plan advocate exercise as an aid to weight reduction and control?

_____ Can your family or living group live with the plan?

_____ Can you live with the diet or a moderate version of the diet for the rest of your life?

If you can answer yes to all of the above questions, you can be reasonably sure you have a good diet plan.

comprise a balanced diet? They should be. It is also important that a wide variety of foods be included. Diets that lack variety get boring quickly and are doomed to failure.

No food is either inherently good or bad for weight loss. Foods used in a successful diet should be inexpensive and easy to acquire. Other family members should be able to eat the same foods, only in larger quantities. A good diet will be one that the dieter can live with forever. Even after the desired weight level is obtained, a modified version of the diet should be used for maintenance. There should be no extravagant promises or guarantees. Weight loss while on the diet should average no more than two pounds per week. Finally, the program should place as much stress on lifelong behavior-modification techniques and exercise as on the diet itself. Successful weight reduction involves a permanent change in life-style, not just a temporary change in diet. The box above is a weight-reduction program evaluation guide. A "yes" answer to all questions on the guide is a sign that the diet program will produce positive results. To be absolutely certain, check with a physician or a dietician.

DIET AIDS

Over-the-counter (OTC) diet aids, those sold in retail stores without a physician's prescription, have become a popular way to support diet and weight-loss programs. It has been estimated that nearly 10 million women in the United States buy OTC diet aids. These aids come in the form of pills, tablets, capsules, powders, milkshakes, and candies. They all work either by reducing the desire to eat or by producing a feeling of fullness that limits the need to eat too much.

The main active ingredient in most over-the-counter diet aids designed to reduce the desire to eat is **phenylpropanolamine (PPA).** This is a controversial drug. Its effects are similar to those

FIGURE 5.1
Over-the-Counter Diet Aids

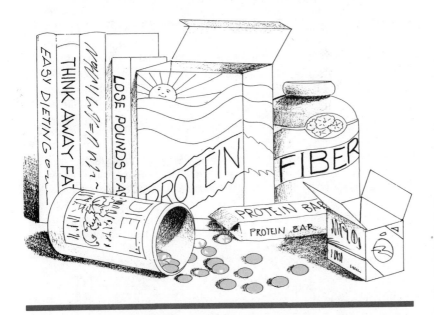

Over-the-counter diet aids come in the form of pills, tablets, capsules, powders, milkshakes, and candies. They all work in one of two ways, either by suppressing the desire to eat (appetite) or by producing a feeling of fullness that encourages the eater to limit his or her food consumption.

Over-the-counter (OTC) diet aid: Any of the variety of products that are promoted as helpful in losing weight and may be purchased without a prescription.

Phenylpropanolamine (PPA): An appetite suppressant used to treat obesity. Prolonged use of this drug can lead to addiction, high blood pressure, nausea, and anxiety.

Did You Know That . . .

*C*al-Ban 3000, advertised as an automatic weight-loss drug, is really guar gum. The gum forms a gel in the stomach that gives a feeling of fullness, but it has no proven benefit for weight reduction.

of **amphetamines**, which raise blood pressure, stimulate the central nervous system, and have the potential for abuse and addiction. While the FDA has found PPA to be safe and effective in the 75-mg dose found in diet aids, critics argue that it is neither safe nor effective.

From the safety perspective, PPA has, as do all drugs, a potential for abuse. Most physicians recommend that PPA as an

(continued on p. 102)

Ten million Americans, mostly women, currently buy diet aids. Since Thompson Medical Company introduced the first over-the-counter diet pill, Dexatrim, in 1977, the number of brands to be found in the local drugstore's "appetite control center" has multiplied steadily. But are they safe for everyone?

The Dish on Diet Aids

How Diet Aids KO Appetite

Although appetite suppressants come in different forms—gums, pills, capsules and tablets—they all work the same way (except for the "natural" fiber products—more about those later). The active ingredient in Dexatrim and most other diet aids is phenylpropanolamine (PPA), which acts on the appetite center in the brain, the hypothalamus, reducing the desire to eat. Found in more than 150 prescription and over-the-counter drugs (including cold medicines and cough syrups), PPA is chemically related to amphetamine. Concerns about this relationship plague PPA's reputation. Critics worry that it mimics the action of amphetamine in susceptible individuals by raising blood pressure, revving up the central nervous system and carrying a potential for abuse and habituation.

When it comes to the 75-mg dose of PPA found in diet aids, some doctors say none of the risks associated with amphetamines apply; others disagree. In 1979, the FDA labeled it a "safe and effective" amount.

A 1985 safety study funded by the Thompson company found that the effects of the 75 mg on pulse and blood pressure in 880 volunteers were not clinically significant. And Jerry Sutkamp, M.D., president of the American Society of Bariatric Physicians, believes that the bad rap PPA diet aids have taken in the past stems from product abuse.

Nevertheless, PPA-related reactions from taking diet aids, including dizziness, heart palpitations, and rapid pulse, have been recently reported to poison-control centers and emergency rooms at a slow but steady rate. Although the incidence of complications is very small, warns Peter Vash, M.D., M.P.H., assistant clinical professor of medicine at the University of California at Los Angeles, PPA "can raise

Amphetamine: A class of drugs that stimulate the nervous system, particularly those that promote the release of chemicals manufactured by the brain (neurotransmitters) that stimulate wakefulness; amphetamines, which are usually available only by prescription, also suppress the appetite and are a common ingredient in many over-the-counter diet aids.

blood pressure and cause cerebral hemorrhaging and strokes—even in some fairly young people."

Public concern over PPA prompted some companies to develop "natural" diet aids—fiber pills and tablets containing no drug. Instead, they suppress your appetite by filling you up with a mixture of grain and citrus fiber. One shouldn't exceed the recommended dosage with these; as one doctor puts it, ingesting more than that is like eating concrete.

The False Promise

All appetite suppressants squelch your appetite, but cannot keep you from choosing fattening goodies when you do eat—so not all dieters drop pounds.

Those who do lose may encounter a different problem. It's recommended that you use PPA-based diet aids for no more than 12 weeks at a time; there is no such time limit for fiber diet aids, but even so, few people envision taking them for life. Once a person stops using a diet aid, she may easily regain the weight.

If You Take Them . . .

If you do decide to use a diet aid with PPA, err on the side of caution: See a physician first to rule out any health risk based on your medical history—even if you only want to lose five pounds. Those who prefer fiber as a filler should know that two and a half tablespoons of bran cereal have the same amount of fiber as a day's dosage of fiber pills.

THE DON'TS OF DIET AIDS

Don't use a diet aid containing PPA if you have

- **high blood pressure**
- **diabetes**
- **thyroid or kidney disease**
- **drug-treated depression**

Discontinue using it if you experience

- **headaches**
- **nervousness**
- **rapid pulse**
- **palpitations**
- **sleeplessness**

Do not use an appetite suppressant with PPA if you are taking another medication—such as cold medicine—containing the substance.

—Liza Galin-Asher

Source: *Mademoiselle* (June 1988), p. 88.

appetite suppressant be consumed for no more than 12 weeks at a time. People successfully losing weight but not yet at their desired weight may be tempted to continue use beyond the recommended time. This could result in a dependence on the drug. Others may attempt to increase the dose to suppress their appetite further, thus increasing their chance of serious side effects. The most common side effects of PPA use are headaches, nervousness, a rapid pulse, heart palpitations, and sleeplessness. Anyone experiencing these symptoms should discontinue use. Further, anyone with high blood pressure, diabetes, thyroid disease, kidney disease, or drug-treated depression should avoid the use of PPA.

The effectiveness of diet aids containing PPA is also in doubt. While they may suppress appetite, they do not influence the types of foods selected for consumption. The dieter may eat less but still eat foods that are high in fats and calories. In this case, the person will lose little or no weight. In addition, when the dieter discontinues the diet aid, he or she will regain any lost weight upon resuming previous eating behaviors.

The second type of diet aid, those that fill up the dieter, are typically composed of grain or citrus fiber. The idea behind these products is that when taken ahead of a meal, they will provide bulk in the stomach so that a feeling of fullness is obtained sooner and the tendency to overeat is reduced. While these products are an alternative for those concerned about using PPA, the result is probably the same. Since most people do not adopt a mind-set to facilitate taking these aids for the rest of their lives, the dieter has not learned any new eating behaviors. When their use is discontinued, he or she will likely go back to the original eating behavior and the lost pounds will, unfortunately, be quickly regained.

SURGICAL SOLUTIONS

Intestinal bypass surgery: A surgical procedure in which a portion of the small intestine is removed and the two ends rejoined thus shortening the overall length of the intestine; while formerly used as a treatment for obesity, this procedure is today most often employed in cancer patients.

Perhaps no weight-control strategy indicates the desperation and despair of the obese more than the various surgical solutions available. These are drastic measures for desperate people. Surgery is costly and may produce serious and painful side effects. For that reason, surgical procedures are only performed on those who are extremely obese and for whom the risk of complications from the surgery is less serious than the risk of complications associated with their obesity.

Intestinal bypass surgery, introduced almost 20 years ago, was the first popular surgical technique. During this procedure, part of the small intestine is disconnected from the digestive tract, leaving a smaller length to do the usual work of digestion. The theory behind this operation is that people inclined to overeat will absorb less of their meals and thus take in fewer calories. This procedure has largely been abandoned because of the serious and life-threatening complications associated with it.

Meanwhile, attention shifted to the stomach. What if the stomach could somehow be made smaller so that the person would feel full more quickly and eat less? To accomplish this, a surgical technique was developed that involved placing a row of surgical staples across the stomach to divide it into two parts. The stomach would then hold less food, and the patient could not eat as much. This procedure has both advocates and critics. It is believed that, with time, the portion of the stomach receiving the food can expand, thus undermining long-term success. In addition, complications, while less severe than those caused by the intestinal surgery, are still a problem. Finally, while people having this surgery do eat less, they also may eat more frequently, and if their food choices are those high in fat and calories, weight loss may still not result.

The next idea for medical intervention in obesity involved placing a balloon in the stomach. The rationale behind this procedure is the same as that for stapling the stomach: If there is less space in the stomach, less can be eaten. The advantage of this procedure is that it does not involve the discomfort and hazards of surgery. The bubble is inserted through an **endoscope**, a tube that can be passed through the mouth into the stomach. A balloon on the end of the endoscope is then blown up to about 200 cubic centimeters, the size of a small grapefruit. The endoscope is then withdrawn, and after a few days of liquid diet, the subject can follow a fairly normal diet. The cost of this procedure, plus diet counseling and training in behavior modification and exercise, is approximately $4,000 to $5,000 a year.

The balloon procedure can cause complications. Constant pressure and the friction of the balloon on the stomach wall increase the risk of developing a stomach ulceration. To minimize the risk of complications, the manufacturer of the balloon recommends that it be left in place no longer than 3 months, although the Food and Drug Administration has approved it for 4 months. Removal of a functioning balloon requires another endoscope procedure. If the balloon should deflate spontaneously, it may pass out of the system with no problem, or it may get trapped in the small intestine, resulting in the need for surgery.

Did You Know That . . .

There are no combinations of foods that burn fat, nor quantities of certain foods (such as eggs or grapefruit) that reduce weight, nor particular times of day when eating is less fattening. These are all persistent diet myths with no validity.

Endoscope: A lighted viewing instrument that can be inserted into a body cavity from the outside allowing visual examination of the interior of the body.

In 1985 the FDA first approved balloons for patients who were 20 percent or more over ideal weight. Because numerous complications were reported, including those listed above, vomiting, and gastric perforations, the FDA readjusted the eligibility standards in 1986 to include only those designated morbidly obese. Further studies have also indicated that the nutritional intake of subjects with balloons is less than adequate. [2]

The crucial question is whether people with the balloon lose weight better than persons without the balloon. To test this, a group of subjects went through the endoscopy procedure. Half were given the balloon and the other half were not. Group members had no idea if they had been given a balloon. Results were not encouraging. In two studies, there were no weight loss differences between those with the balloon and those without. In a third study, the balloon group demonstrated a modest advantage over the non-balloon group in the first 4 months of the study, but during a subsequent 4-month period, there were no differences between groups.

Another method for weight loss involves wiring the jaw shut for a period of time. The idea here is that the patient will be forced to follow a liquid diet and will lose weight. Although weight loss usually occurs with this procedure, the long-term results are not encouraging. Most persons gain back the weight when they return to normal eating behaviors. [3]

A final type of medical intervention, **liposuction**, also deserves mention. This is really a cosmetic surgery approach to weight control. If the person cannot lose the weight, it will be surgically removed through a suction device. While this technique has appeal in that it produces very quick results, it obviously does nothing to deal with the way a person eats, stores, and burns calories. Lifelong dietary and exercise changes must be implemented if the weight is to be kept off.

LIQUID DIETS

The latest weight-loss procedure to receive significant attention by the media and medical community is the liquid diet, known as the **very-low-calorie diet (VLCD)**. Popularized by talk-show host Oprah Winfrey, who lost 67 pounds on such a diet, more than 450 diets like hers are offered throughout the country. As many as 2,000 hospitals offer similar types of programs. Essentially, a VLCD program involves going on a *medically supervised,* modified fast for up to 12 weeks. During this time, the only food eaten

Liposuction: A surgical technique in which excess adipose tissue (storage fat) beneath the skin is removed by a suction device; also known as suction lipectomy.

Very-low-calorie diet (VLCD): A medically supervised diet wherein the patient fasts for up to 12 weeks on food consisting of a powder formula mixed with water that provides essential nutrients while supplying only 400 to 600 calories per day.

is a powder formula mixed with water. It provides essential nutrients to prevent deficiencies from occurring, while only 400 to 600 calories are consumed per day. Once the fasting portion is completed, foods are reintroduced and behavior-modification techniques are taught.

Current VLCDs are significantly different from the liquid-protein diets first introduced two decades ago. The earlier versions were available over the counter, were not medically supervised, and were nutritionally inadequate. More than 50 deaths were associated with use of OTC liquid-protein diet products. Today's VLCDs are available only through medically supervised programs, have improved nutritional quality, and are considered far safer than the earlier liquid formulas. This does not mean there are no risks associated with today's liquid diets. While health problems associated with VLCDs are neither as severe nor life-threatening as were those associated with earlier liquid-protein diets, they still exist. Some patients experience physical problems such as dizziness, fainting, constipation, diarrhea, dry skin, and hair loss. There are no figures on how many VLCD clients experience these symptoms, but few experts deny that such problems exist.

Furthermore, VLCDs are not for everyone and can be harmful for persons who:

1. Are not at least 30 percent overweight, with a minimum body mass index of 32

2. Are pregnant or suffering from any of the following medical complications: cancer, liver disease, kidney failure, active cardiac dysfunction, or severe psychological disturbances

3. Are not committed to establishing new eating and life-style behaviors that will assist the maintenance of weight loss

4. Are not committed to taking the time to complete both the treatment and maintenance components of a diet program [4]

Above all, one should never attempt a VLCD diet without medical supervision. It is the position of the American Dietetic Association that "while very-low-calorie diets promote rapid weight loss and may be beneficial for certain individuals, such diets have health risks and should be undertaken only with the supervision of a multidisciplinary health team with monitoring by a physician and nutrition counseling by a registered dietician." [5]

Did You Know That . . .

During 1990, some 65 million Americans spent more than $32 billion on products related to weight control.

Once eligibility is established, a candidate must undergo a complete medical examination before being allowed to enter the program. Some programs require candidates to adopt a weight-stabilizing diet or take a course in behavior modification before starting the VLCD. The cost of these programs is also restrictive. Reportedly, it takes $100–$150 a week to be on the VLCD, with the total cost of the program averaging $2,500. [6] Compounding the cost problem is the fact that most major insurance companies do not cover VLCDs. Therefore, these programs are out of reach for many Americans.

The drop-out rate for VLCD programs is also very high. It is estimated that 30 to 55 percent of those entering a VLCD program will drop out before completing the program. An even greater problem involves maintaining weight once the fast is completed. During the fast, people typically report little or no feeling of hunger. They know they are allowed only the liquid formula and have no food choices to make. Once off the fast phase, however, people are again faced with food selections and old patterns are easily reestablished. In one 30-month study of 2,200 patients conducted by Kaiser Permanente Medical Group in San Diego, California, 40 percent of those completing the program had regained nearly all the weight they had lost. Some even gained more. The remaining 60 percent of the patients had regained an average of 40 percent of their initial loss. [7]

While the success rates for VLCD programs may not seem impressive, they are certainly better than the 5- to 10-percent success rates typically reported in other weight programs for the obese. There is little doubt that these liquid formula diets, when properly supervised, can help the severely obese to lose weight. By most standards, they also would be considered safer and more reasonable than the various surgical alternatives. It must be remembered, however, that the quick fix offered by VLCD programs is only as effective as the behavior-modification techniques and ultimate life-style changes that must occur after the weight is lost. There is no such thing as a quick, easy, permanent weight-loss method.

The newest attempt to help Americans reduce weight and improve health are **fat substitutes**, the "fake fats." The Food and Drug Administration recently approved the first fat substitute, Nutrasweet's Simplesse, and several additional such substitutes are pending approval. Simplesse is made of proteins from egg whites and milk; Nutrasweet labels it "all natural." So far, the FDA has allowed its use only in frozen desserts, but it soon may also be approved for mayonnaise, salad dressings, sour cream,

Fat substitute: A food product designed to simulate the taste and texture of animal or vegetable fat while containing fewer calories.

(continued on p. 108)

FIGURE 5.2
Fat Substitutes

A. Fat Content in Traditional Foods vs. Foods Containing Fat Substitutes

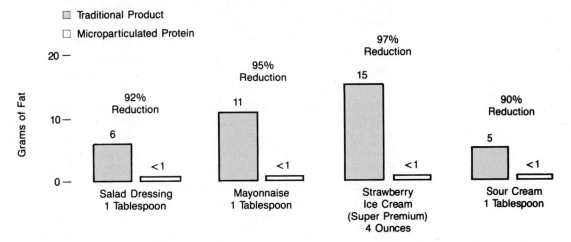

B. Calorie Content in Traditional Foods vs. Foods Containing Fat Substitutes

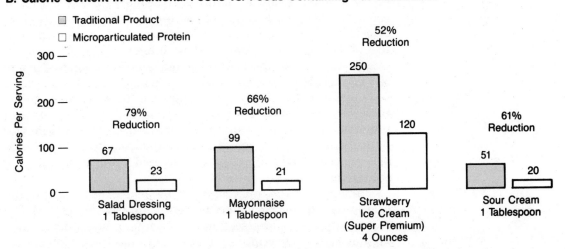

Source: Nutritive Value of American Foods in Common Units, USDA, Agricultural Handbook No. 8, Washington, DC, (8-1), 1976; (8-4), 1979. Information on File, Hazleton Labs, Madison, WI, 1989.

Fat substitutes are made from microparticulated protein. **A** shows the fat content in certain foods and in foods containing fat substitutes, while **B** shows that fat substitutes not only reduce fat intake but also contain fewer calories.

and cheese spreads. Simplesse does have two drawbacks. It cannot be used in any product that will be heated because it coagulates (gels) at high temperatures. Also, people allergic to eggs or milk may be allergic to this fat substitute, which contains them. [8]

Since fats are a bigger problem for most Americans than sugars when it comes to weight control, fake fats could become an even bigger business than artificial sweeteners. The Calorie Control Council, an international association of manufacturers of low-calorie and diet foods and beverages, has made projections of the potential impact of fat substitutes. The actual impact of these new fat substitutes, however, is yet to be seen. [9]

SPAS

The **spa**, or live-in weight-loss clinic (sometimes called a fat farm), is another option open to those with large bank accounts. Such clinics are quite popular among the rich and famous. Essentially, a live-in clinic structures the life of the patient in such a way that weight loss will occur. Exercise is a main component of most clinic programs. Long walks, aerobic dance, swimming, water exercising, and other types of physical exercise are interwoven into the day's activities. Meals, although expertly prepared and presented, usually provide only 600 to 800 calories per day. Under these conditions of high-caloric output and low-caloric input, all but the most difficult cases will lose weight over the 1-month period typical for these clinics.

In addition to the rigid diet and exercise program, live-in clinics include a generous amount of pampering in the form of body massage, hot tubs, saunas, and even "herbal wraps." While these services contribute nothing to losing body fat, they do make the diet and exercise seem more bearable. Classes in behavior modification, cooking, stress management, and beauty aids are also typical. Many of the clinics are located in warm climates and the surroundings are quite plush.

A recent article in *Changing Times* magazine identified and briefly described 12 popular live-in weight-loss clinics. [10] The cost to attend a 4-week session ranged from a low of $2,000 to a high of $7,187. Descriptions of the clinics also varied considerably. Some focused on the spa-like pampering and famous stars who had previously attended the clinic, while others emphasized the medical supervision and scientific approach to weight loss.

Do fat farms really reduce body fat? The answer to this question is probably yes. After all, if a person is given only

Spa: An often luxurious, residential, resort-like facility that is operated on a commercial basis and offers a variety of health-related services including weight-reduction programs.

"SUPERSTARS' DIET SECRETS! Shed pounds the rich-and-famous way!" shouts the headline. Your hand reaches out. How *did* Liz . . .

Forget it. There are no tricks, no secrets, no miracles. The people who succeed at losing weight are the ones who see through the hokum and false promises. Here are seven matters of fat you ought to know.

DIET AIDS DON'T WORK. Over-the-counter appetite suppressants contain

Matters of Fat

the decongestant phenylpropanolamine, or PPA, which disrupts hunger signals to the brain and dries out the mouth, making food taste bland and unappetizing. Side effects can include nervousness, irritability, insomnia, and high blood pressure.

If you don't mind chewing tasteless food and living with a bad disposition, such products *can* curb your appetite, but not for long. Once you're off the pills, a step that's medically advisable after three months, any weight you lost will probably sneak right back.

Diet chewing gums and candy, to be taken before meals, are more benign—but less helpful. They contain benzocaine, which numbs the mouth's nerve endings, making them less sensitive to sweet. You'll keep your taste for fat.

DIET SODAS MAY NOT HELP. Though one study did actually show that artificial-sweetener users consumed 165 fewer calories a day, another found that women using such sweeteners were even *more* likely to gain weight than those who didn't. Many people save 30 or so calories by stirring a packet of artificial sweetener into their after-dinner coffee, then use that virtue as an excuse to order chocolate mousse.

THERE'S NO SUCH THING AS CELLULITE. The orange-peel dimpling that often occurs around women's thighs and hips is just plain, ordinary fat. Strands of tissue near the skin separate fat compartments and anchor them to deeper muscles. When these fat cells are extremely full they bulge, leaving little valleys—the "cellulite"—in between. Skip the loofah sponges, the horsehair mitts, and other touted remedies. The way to get rid of the dimples is to lose weight, preferably before age 35 or 40, when your skin is still elastic enough to shrink back.

YOU CAN'T SLIM JUST ONE BODY PART. Do leg-lifts and you may burn enough calories to lose some fat, but not necessarily from around your thighs. In fact, by toning the muscles beneath a layer of fat, they could make your legs even bigger. Only good old aerobic exercise, sustained for 15 or 20 minutes, melts body fat. Rubberized sweatsuits, sauna belts, and cellophane wraps simply dehydrate you.

The one real treatment for localized fat is liposuction, a surgical process that removes fat cells from under the skin. It's expensive, risky, and sometimes painful.

YOU CAN'T LOSE WEIGHT FOREVER. On most diets the first few pounds come off quickly because less food means fewer carbohydrates and less salt—both of which lead to water losses. At the same time metabolism slows. Plus, as more weight comes off, you spend less energy to move. For every 25-pound drop, you need 100 fewer calories a day. To keep losing weight, keep upping your exercise.

SOME PEOPLE ARE BORN TO BE THIN. It's not fair, but when it comes to metabolic rates, we're not all created equal. In general, metabolic rates are faster in infants, adolescents, and pregnant women; in men, who typically have more muscle than women; and in tall, thin people, whose larger surface area radiates more heat. Even when two people are the same sex, height, and weight, one's metabolism may burn 1,400 a day, the other person's 1,000. No one knows why.

EVERYBODY GETS FATTER WITH AGE. Between the ages of 20 and 50, the typical body both adds fat and loses muscle. The fat content of a man's body usually doubles, while a woman's increases by half. It happens because the metabolism slows by two percent each decade; and unless you maintain or increase your activity level, you'll inevitably get fatter. A small weight gain may not be bad. Some evidence suggests that people who *slowly* gain weight with age may not be adding to their risk of disease or premature death.

Source: Patricia Long, *Hippocrates* (September/October 1989), p. 45.

prescribed portions of food and is required to increase his or her exercise levels, reducing body fat is not that difficult. A better question to ask is, "Do fat farms help people keep the excess pounds off?" The answer to this question is not as clear. Long-term weight-loss statistics were not presented for any live-in clinics. It is certainly appropriate to question if a person will be motivated to follow the same diet and exercise program once the structure of the live-in environment is no longer present.

THE CELLULITE MYTH

Cellulite: Popular name for lumpy, dimpled fat deposits, particularly those sometimes found on the thighs and buttocks; experts agree that there is no difference between "cellulite" and other fatty deposits.

Popular notion has it that the unsightly dimpled fat that often occurs around women's thighs and hips is a special type of fat called **cellulite**. Supposedly, cellulite is more difficult to eliminate than regular fat and requires special types of treatment. As a result, a host of products have been developed to deal with this problem. In actuality, however, *there is no such thing as cellulite.*

The dimpled fat is just plain ordinary fat. Strands of tissue near the skin separate fat into compartments and attach themselves to deeper tissue layers. When the fat compartments are full, they bulge, leaving little valleys where the attachments occurred. The only way to lose these dimples is to lose weight, preferably before the age of 35 or 40, through a balanced program that reduces your overall weight. The horsehair mitts and other remedies will do little to remove the undesirable dimples.

The mark of any effective weight-loss program is not how much is lost in the first week, first month, or even the first 6 months. It is how much body fat one has 1, 2, and 3 years after the start of the program. Too often, we Americans are concerned with the quick fix. We do not seem to realize the extra pounds that may

Did You Know That . . .

Cellulite may not be a special kind of fat, but emollients to smooth the skin and massage to break up fat clumps may alleviate the dimpled look.

FIGURE 5.3
Fat Is Fat

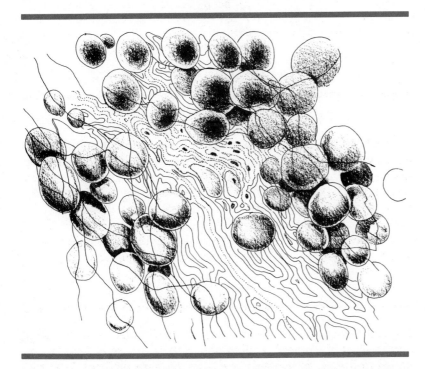

This drawing shows subcutaneous fat cells, connective tissue, and muscle fiber. The dimpled fat that often occurs around women's thighs and hips, popularly known as cellulite, is only normal bulging fat cells admidst strands of tissue. The only way to lose these dimples is to lose weight.

have taken years to put on are going to take months and even years to take off. The desire for quick results makes people vulnerable to fads and gimmicks that at best don't work and at worst may be physically harmful while costing considerable amounts of money.

In addition to the problems associated with taking excess weight off, there is the problem of keeping it off. There seems to be little recognition among average Americans that weight control is a lifelong commitment. If you have become overweight as a result of your current eating habits, those habits can never be followed again without gaining weight. However, we often hear people talk about dieting as though it is a temporary inconvenience, a set of goals that entails dieting only until we are able to fit into a certain size of clothes.

Once again, avoid all fads, gimmicks, gadgets, and any weight-reduction program claiming to produce fast, easy weight loss. For most people, the best way to lose weight and keep it off is to combine a sensible, balanced diet with an appropriate exercise program and to recognize that a lifelong change in eating behavior is necessary. [W]

Other Weight-Related Problems

C H A P T E R

6

ALTHOUGH MOST OF THE ATTENTION in our society goes to those who are obese, there are significant numbers of people who are underweight. **Underweight** is defined as being 10 percent or more under the ideal weight as indicated by the height and weight charts. For these individuals, the trials and tribulations of trying to gain weight can be just as frustrating as attempts to lose weight are for the overfat person.

UNDERWEIGHT

The health hazards of being underweight are neither well understood nor agreed upon. Some experts believe that **life expectancy** decreases for those people 10 percent or more below ideal body weight, just as it does for overfat people. Other experts attribute the decrease in longevity of underweight people to higher rates of cigarette smoking and chronic disease, both of which may cause decreased body weight. Additional research is needed before we can make more definitive statements regarding the health effects of being underweight.

The first step for the underweight individual is to see his or her physician to rule out the possibility of an underlying physical problem contributing to or causing the underweight condition. This is especially important if there has been an unexplained or rapid loss of weight. Once it has been determined that the underweight individual is essentially healthy, counting calories, increasing high-calorie food consumption, eating regular meals, and adding a fourth meal just before bedtime may help to

Underweight: A statistical designation based on total body weight which is 10 percent or more under the ideal weight indicated on a standard height and weight chart.

Life expectancy: The average number of years remaining in the life of a living being, it can be predicted at any time in the life of the being by averaging the age at death of all members of the species over a fixed period of time.

increase weight. Exercise should not be discontinued in an attempt to reduce caloric expenditure to facilitate weight gain. Muscle tone and conditioning levels need to be maintained regardless of one's weight. For someone engaged in intense training, however, the amount of exercise may be reduced. As with obesity, it is best not to expect immediate results and to modify weight slowly over time. A most unfortunate way to solve one's problem of being underweight is to become obese instead.

COLLEGE FEMALES AND NEGATIVE FOOD ATTITUDES

College campuses are a perfect breeding ground for **eating disorders**, or dieting behavior harmful to one's health. College students are often away from home for the first time and have no real supervision over their eating behaviors. Sit-down meals are no longer required, while vending machines and fast-food establishments abound. Unfortunately, an eating disorder is easy to conceal. It is easy for a college student to tell friends or roommates that he or she has already grabbed a bite. In an unstructured environment, no one will know the difference.

The actual number of women suffering from eating disorders depends upon how rigorous one's definition of "eating disorder" is.

Eating disorder: A chronic pattern of abnormal dieting behavior that has negative health effects; the 2 best known eating disorders are anorexia nervosa and bulimia.

The Majorette Diet

You'd expect big-time college football players to have health problems, from blown knees to the side effects of steroids. But the majorettes on the sidelines may be even more at risk—from the unsafe diet they follow to meet arbitrary weight requirements set by their faculty advisers.

So finds one study published in *The Physician and Sports Medicine*. Researchers interviewed 11 varsity majorettes from a large midwestern university at the beginning of the last football season. They asked the majorettes what they had eaten in the last 24 hours and what their dieting methods were. The women were reinterviewed during the football season.

All of the majorettes had distorted body images. Despite evidence to the contrary, they thought they were fat. They were chronic dieters. The women, who averaged just under 20 years of age, expended a great deal of energy during practices, yet survived on a paltry 690 to 1,100 calories a day.

Their diets were deficient in protein, iron, calcium, potassium and, of course, calories. Of the 11 majorettes, four had menstrual irregularities, one was chronically constipated and one fainted after a low-intensity fitness test. The woman who fainted—with a slight 112 lb. on her 5'5" frame—hadn't eaten or even drunk water in 36 hours. Her major: health sciences.

How did these women get that way? Much of the blame rests with their faculty adviser, as well as peer pressure and poor role models, the study finds. The majorettes, who were required to meet the adviser's arbitrary weight standards, would sit in saunas, take diet pills, exercise heavily and avoid food for up to two days. They were made to weigh in publicly once a week, a couple of days before the football game. If a majorette didn't make her weight, she was replaced for that game—a humiliating experience. The majorettes who made their weights would often then indulge in binge eating (and vomiting).

It's a classic example of psychological conditioning, notes study co-author and psychiatrist Laurie L. Humphries at the University of Kentucky. With an adviser acting as an authority figure, she says, the women are encouraged to believe they are too fat. In this way, their unhealthy behavior is rewarded.

Many of the majorettes said they wanted to change these long-reinforced habits—some had been on diets since they were eight years old—but they felt trapped between their desire for sensible nutrition and pressure applied by the faculty adviser and peers.

Despite Dr. Humphries's efforts, the adviser has shown no willingness to help these students. Instead of giving the majorettes access to nutritional counseling, a "diet specialist" has been hired from a local weight-loss clinic.

—*Kevin Cobb*

Source: *American Health* (December 1988), p. 95.

Did You Know That . . .

Overzealous dieting by adolescents can lead to "nutritional dwarfing"—a slow or halted growth rate. To develop normally, youngsters need more calories, fat, and carbohydrates than their parents do.

Using stricter definitions, estimates have been as low as 1 to 3 percent. With less rigorous definitions, the estimated prevalence of eating disorders among young women has been as high as 20 percent. [1] Eating disorders are not limited to the anonymous college student. Recently, Megan Neyer, a world-class diver, was reportedly suffering eating disorders. [2] Other female athletes, particularly gymnasts and distance runners, seem prone to them. Athletes are especially susceptible since they face the pressure of competition combined with the pressure to maintain a specific body build.

Even if a young woman does not have a full-blown eating disorder, negative mental attitudes regarding eating, body image, and weight control have become the norm rather than the excep-

Table 6.1 Risk Factors for Developing an Eating Disorder

Individual

- Autonomy, identity and separation concerns
- Perceptual disturbances
- Weight preoccupation
- Cognitive disturbances
- Chronic medical illnesses (insulin-dependent diabetes)

Family

- Inherited biological predisposition
  —family history of eating disorders
  —family history of alcoholism, affective illness
  —family history of obesity (bulimia)
- Magnification of cultural factors
- Parent-child interactions leading to problems with autonomy
  and separation

Cultural

- Pressures for thinness
- Pressures for performance

Source: National Institute on Nutrition, "An Overview of the Eating Disorders Anorexia Nervosa and Bulimia Nervosa," *Nutrition Today* (May/June 1989), p. 28.

Risk factors for anorexia nervosa and bulimia nervosa. The two diseases are similar in that they involve a dramatic preoccupation with body weight. Anorexics exhibit this obsession through self-starvation, whereas bulimics do so by rapidly consuming and then vomiting large quantities of food, or "binging and purging."

tion among female college students. The problem is so great that it prompted the director of women's studies at Cornell University to state that "college students today are more promiscuous about food than they are about sex." [3] In a 1984 study of 192 female college students, 82 percent wanted to lose weight, although only 8 percent were actually overweight. Of the group desiring unnecessary weight loss:

- Laxative abuse was reported by 8.3 percent.
- Intentionally induced vomiting had been used by 13.5 percent.
- Diuretics had been abused by 14.6 percent.
- Diets of 800 calories or less had been followed by 39 percent.

Furthermore, 62 percent of this population reported uncontrollable urges to eat. It is interesting to note that the more negative the subjects' attitudes were toward food, the greater the number of hazardous weight-control behaviors they practiced. This was true regardless of the subjects' weight status. [4]

These data are not just shocking, they are frightening. They clearly demonstrate the extent of eating-related problems for college women. The results strongly support the need for good nutrition education and counseling services for college-age female students. While the prevalence of eating disorders among college males is not nearly as high as for college females, males are nonetheless susceptible. Estimates for college males suffering eating disorders range from 0.1 percent to 5 percent. [5]

ANOREXIA NERVOSA

Anorexia nervosa, a refusal to eat or a severely abnormal eating pattern, is an eating disorder most commonly found among young women. It is generally agreed that the prevalence of anorexia is increasing. According to recent estimates, 1 out of every 200 (0.5 percent) American girls between the ages of 12 and 18 will develop anorexia nervosa to some degree. [6] The disorder is characterized by a relentless pursuit of thinness, coupled with an exaggerated fear of weight gain. Anorexics have a severely

(continued on p. 119)

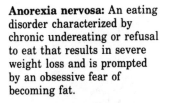

Table 6.2 Early Signs of Anorexia Nervosa and Bulimia Nervosa

- Changing weight goals
- Dieting that leads to increasing criticism of one's body
- Dieting that leads to social isolation
- Loss of menstrual periods
- Hiding foods, vomiting, misuse of laxatives, diuretics and diet pills

Source: National Institute on Nutrition, "An Overview of the Eating Disorders Anorexia Nervosa and Bulimia Nervosa," *Nutrition Today* (May/June 1989), p. 28.

Some symptoms of eating disorders, which have become increasingly prevalent on college campuses and among high school students during recent years.

Anorexia nervosa: An eating disorder characterized by chronic undereating or refusal to eat that results in severe weight loss and is prompted by an obsessive fear of becoming fat.

FIGURE 6.1
Anorexia Nervosa and Self-Image

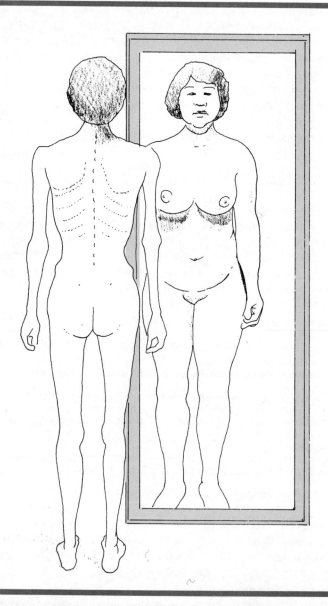

Those who suffer from anorexia nervosa (anorexics) have a distorted self-image. Even when they have become dangerously thin from excessive dieting, they see themselves as too fat.

Table 6.3 Common Signs and Symptoms of Starvation

Physical

Dry skin
Soft, downy hair on body
Brittle nails
Yellow skin
Low heart rate
Low blood pressure
Bloating
Constipation
Early satiety
Cessation of menstrual
  cycle
Low blood sugar

Low blood potassium
Reduced body temperature
Stunting of growth
Susceptibility to bone
  fracture

Psychological

Food preoccupation
Depressed mood
Irritable mood
Diminished libido
Broken sleep

Source: Adapted from National Institute on Nutrition, "An Overview of the Eating Disorders Anorexia Nervosa and Bulimia Nervosa," *Nutrition Today* (May/June 1989), p. 28.

Anorexics in the advanced stages of the disease become victims of starvation and suffer some or all of its symptoms. At this stage prompt medical attention is required, or the consequences can be fatal.

distorted self-image. Despite being excessively and unattractively thin, they think they look fat. They often identify specific body parts as being too large. They do not perceive their dietary behavior as abnormal and do not wish to change it. Above all else, they do not want to gain weight. Mastery and control of dietary intake become central issues for anorexics. They take pride in their ability to restrict calories and often see dieting as one area of their lives in which they are a success.

The physical symptoms of anorexia are a direct product of starvation. Anorexic bodies appear to be skin and bones. Feminine curves have disappeared and clothes just seem to hang. In addition, anorexics often have dry, cracking skin and may be losing scalp hair. Hands and feet are usually cold and blue in color. **Bradycardia** (low heart rate), **hypotension** (low blood pressure), and low body temperature may be evident. Patients who induce vomiting to restrict calories further may suffer various dental problems.

When anorexics first start to diet, their initial goal is just to lose a few pounds. They usually start by cutting out sweets, desserts, and high-calorie snacks. As a result of their success with

(continued on p. 121)

Did You Know That . . .

In a study of 271 adolescent girls, nearly 50 percent perceived themselves as too fat. By contrast, the researchers found, 83 percent of the subjects were actually of normal weight.

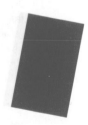

Bradycardia: An abnormally low heart rate (less than 60 beats per minute in an adult); bradycardia may or may not be an indicator of an underlying disorder.

Hypotension: The medical term for abnormally low blood pressure.

The Resurgence of Anorexia

Can history help us come to grips with one of the most devastating emotional disorders of modern young women, the self-imposed starvation that is the hallmark of anorexia nervosa?

Yes, says Dr. Joan Jacobs Brumberg, author of "Fasting Girls: The Emergence of Anorexia Nervosa as a Modern Disease" (Harvard University Press). A historical perspective, she insists, can both help us to understand the origins of eating disorders and suggest guidelines for stemming the current epidemic, which Dr. Brumberg believes has not yet reached its peak.

Anorexia nervosa is not a new disease, said Dr. Brumberg, who is director of women's studies as well as associate professor of human development and family studies at Cornell University. The disease did not emerge with the fashion industry's focus on emaciated female bodies, although the modern imperative to be thin is feeding the epidemic of eating disorders. Although no precise statistics exist, an estimated 10 percent of American women have eating disorders, including anorexia, and on college campuses the number often exceeds 20 percent, she said.

Dr. Brumberg demonstrates that women have been fasting for various reasons at least since medieval times, when some young women starved themselves in a quest for religious perfection. It resurfaced in a more secular form in Victorian times. At that time, changes in family and social dynamics, especially the emergence of a bourgeois class that treated young girls and women as delicate creatures, put pressure on privileged women to deny their appetites for food, which they tended to equate with an appetite for sex.

Anorexia nervosa, meaning emotionally caused loss of appetite, was first identified by physicians in England, France and the United States in the 1870's, long before any modern preoccupation with dieting.

But not until after World War II did the incidence of anorexia begin to rise, under the combined influences of growing affluence, greater availability of food, increased expectations for achievement and rising social pressures on young women. And not until the 1970's did it take off, receiving the attention that led to both a greater likelihood of diagnosis and a significant increase in the number of girls who learned about anorexia and "chose" it to express their emotional and social turmoil.

Any theory about the underlying causes of anorexia must take into account characteristics of the disease that have prevailed since at least the mid-19th century. Dr. Brumberg said that anorexia is prevalent only in affluent societies when the economy is thriving. The incidence was very low in the Depression and World War II.

It is a syndrome almost exclusively limited to adolescent girls and young women from middle- and upper-class families. Although some young men develop anorexia, 90 to 95 percent of current victims are women or girls. Victims of anorexia are nearly always conscientious, hardworking, dependable overachievers who were trouble-free until they got sick.

"Today there is a whole new set of stresses that are added to the ordinary sexual pressures on young women," Dr. Brumberg said in an interview. "We have raised women's expectations without giving them adequate social support. They are fearful about many things: integrating career and family, changes in sex and gender roles, sexually transmitted diseases, commitment, family instability as evidenced by the high rates of divorce."

It is not surprising, then, that so many young women develop a disease that strips them of their sexuality and physical maturity. Dr. Brumberg also sees anorexia as "a perfect psychopathology" for the "Superwoman" of the 1970's and 80's.

"For the modern woman, being thin is the ultimate form of perfection," she wrote. "The kind of personal control required to become the new

Superwoman parallels the single-mindedness that characterizes the anorectic."

Overemphasis on Beauty

Dr. Brumberg views anorexia as a "secular addiction to a new kind of perfectionism, one that links personal salvation to the achievement of an external body configuration rather than an internal spiritual state."

But the biggest push has come from society's overemphasis on beauty and a degree of slimness that is abnormal for most women, combined with the constant availability of tempting foods.

Dr. Brumberg sees college campuses as the perfect breeding grounds for eating disorders.

"There are no required sit-down meals anymore," she said. "Students today eat everywhere, every hour of the day and almost anything you can imagine." Everywhere a student turns, there are vending machines, delis and fast-food establishments, some of which will even deliver in the middle of the night.

"For a youngster prone to an eating disorder, it can be an extraordinary struggle to stick to an eating pattern," Dr. Brumberg said, adding that "college students today are more promiscuous about food than they are about sex."

Since millions of young women are exposed to the same cultural conditions, why don't many more develop anorexia? Clearly, Dr. Brumberg said, cultural pressures alone do not cause the disorder. Rather, culture interacts with individual psychology, biology and family influences, resulting in an "addiction to starvation" among vulnerable women.

Fighting the Epidemic

How can the epidemic of eating disorders be stemmed? As a historian and feminist, Dr. Brumberg supports efforts to foster emotional and social development of women, some of which have already taken root. Among other things, she suggests the following:

• More emphasis should be put on intellectual activities and creativity.

• Women's magazines, which promote an endless stream of weight-loss plans and beauty makeovers, should place less emphasis on the social presentation of self.

• Society should not be afraid to extol the more traditional virtues of women as feeling, caring, healing beings. In the process of rejecting sexist stereotypes, society has de-emphasized these attributes and fails to present them to young women as a source of satisfaction.

"I'm not suggesting that women should pay no attention to their physical well-being," she said. "We should all try to eat healthfully and keep ourselves physically fit. But we have to lose that intense preoccupation with the external body as the be-all and end-all of a woman's worth."

Source: Jane E. Brody, "Personal Health," *New York Times*, 19 May 1988, sec. 2, p. 14.

this generally healthy behavioral change, they may receive praise and recognition from friends and family. The praise and recognition encourage them to restrict their diets further and further until they may be eating only 600 to 800 calories per day. As time passes, they begin to fear foods, particularly high-carbohydrate foods that they perceive may induce weight gain. The list of acceptable foods decreases until the only acceptable items are cottage cheese, salads, vegetables, and fruit. Some victims will eat exactly the same foods every day for months at a time.

FIGURE 6.2
Anorexia Nervosa in Earlier Times

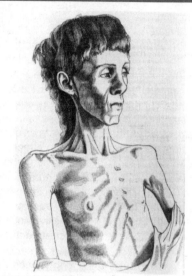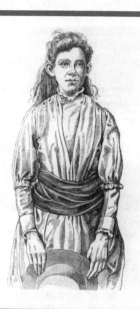

Source: National Library of Medicine.

The changing role of women in the Victorian era made women vulnerable to eating disorders. Shown here is a young woman who suffered from anorexia nervosa and whose case was first reported in 1888. After six months of treatment, she recovered fully.

Eventually, as friends and relatives become concerned with the extreme weight loss, pressure may be placed on the anorexic to eat more. As a result, she will often adopt deceptive behaviors. She may secretly feed her food to the dog, flush a meal down the toilet, or throw it in the garbage. She may tell parents and friends that she has already eaten or that she is not hungry. Some anorexics will vomit after meals to keep the food from being digested. Others will abuse laxatives for the same purpose.

"Anorexia" literally means lack of appetite, but this does not happen until late in the starvation process. Often aware of hunger, the anorexic will overcome this sensation through her extreme fear of becoming fat. Because of hunger, some are driven to consume appetite suppressants, such as amphetamines or diet pills. Some drink large quantities of fluid to feel full. Still others will interpret their feelings of hunger as a positive sign of self-control. With time, even when food is eaten, satiety perception (the feeling of fullness) becomes extremely distorted. Small quantities of food produce feelings of distension and bloating.

Another common feature of anorexic behavior is excessive exercise. Exercise is initially used to reduce calories further. As with dieting, however, the exercise may soon become a further sign of self-control for the patient. It may become extremely compulsive, with anorexics refusing to miss even one day of workouts for fear of gaining weight and losing control.

Most anorexics gradually narrow their interests and withdraw. They may eventually restrict activities only to dieting, exercise, and school work. Everything else falls by the wayside. As the disease progresses, anorexics may become depressed, lose all interest in sexuality, and go out of their way to avoid encounters with the opposite sex. Ego and self-esteem drop; anorexics often begin mistrusting themselves, their impulses, and their feelings.

This is not a pleasant picture, and the long-term prospects for recovery are not good, either. Overall, studies indicate about 40 percent of those diagnosed as anorexic recover under treatment and an additional 30 percent show "significant improvement." The remaining 30 percent make little or no improvement. Mortality rates from various studies range from 0 to 24 percent, with the average being around 9 percent. The prognosis for recovery seems to improve if the victim is relatively young at the age of onset, is from a middle- or upper-class family, does not practice force vomiting, and has previously performed well at school and work. The average interval required to re-establish normal body weight is 3 years, but this interval can extend to 5 years or more. [7]

BULIMIA

Bulimia, also called bulimia nervosa, bulimarexia, and dietary chaos syndrome, is defined as "recurrent episodes of rapid uncontrollable ingestion of large amounts of food in a short period of time, usually followed by purging either by forced vomiting and/or abuse of laxatives or diuretics." [8] This is commonly known as "binge and purge." Although bulimia is actually an eating disorder in its own right, 30 to 50 percent of anorexics also binge and purge. Bulimia can affect women at any time from the teens to middle age. The most vulnerable, however, are white middle-class adolescents and women in their twenties who are academically oriented and desire a traditional life-style, including marriage.

Bulimia: An eating disorder characterized by ingesting large amounts of food over a short period of time, followed by forced vomiting to avoid weight gain.

Many are intelligent, physically attractive, and capable of handling stressful careers. Despite these positive qualities, they typically have abnormally low self-esteem, a desire for perfection, a sense of loneliness and isolation, and an obsession with food and body weight.

While a greater percentage of females exhibit one or two symptoms of bulimia, it is more rare to find women who possess all the symptoms of clinical bulimia nervosa. These symptoms include:

- Recurrent episodes of binge eating (rapid consumption of a large amount of food in a limited period of time, usually less than 2 hours)
- Fear of being unable to stop eating during eating binges
- Engaging in either self-induced vomiting, laxative use, or rigorous dieting or fasting in order to counteract the effects of binge eating
- A minimum average of two binge-eating episodes per week for at least 3 months [9]

Experts estimate that 2 to 5 percent of all adolescent and young adult females suffer bulimia. [10]

Bulimics usually have average-to-thin body builds by any standard except their own. They invariably feel fat and regard their bodies far more critically than so-called "normal women." They are perfectionists and their bodies are never right. Their breasts are too small, their thighs too big or hips too pronounced, and so forth.

There are some similarities between bulimia and anorexia nervosa. Both anorexics and bulimics are likely to have been brought up in middle-class, upwardly mobile families. In such families, mothers usually are too involved in their daughter's lives and fathers are preoccupied with work outside the home. Both anorexics and bulimics are typically "good children," eager to comply and to achieve so as to obtain the love and recognition of others.

But significant differences also exist between anorexics and bulimics. Bulimics are usually of normal weight or slightly overweight, whereas anorexics are extremely underweight. Anorexics are generally younger, less socially competent, and much more isolated from and yet dependent on the family. The health of bulimics may be affected by their behavior, but their lives are usually not in danger, as an anorexic's is. Biochemical changes that result from the anorexic's self-starvation typically cause both

(continued on p. 127)

Psychologic Treatment for Binge Eating

Many of us overeat from time to time. In most cases we are apt to forgive ourselves, perhaps vowing not to overeat the next time. Often we will attribute our overeating to the palatability of the food, reasoning that it tasted so good that we simply had difficulty stopping. However, binge eating, or bulimia, is a problem that is distinct from overeating and frequently leads to serious physical and psychologic difficulties. The characteristics that distinguish a binge from an episode of overeating are the following: (1) the food is consumed within a relatively brief period of time and (2) the person experiences a loss of control during the episode. People with bulimia frequently report negative emotional reactions after binges. Depression, guilt, and self-denigration are common. Binge eating usually occurs secretly and often involves the consumption of high-calorie food. The behavior has a driven, or compulsive, quality to it, and bulimics often report that they do not really taste or enjoy the food once a binge is under way.

Binge eating is a feature of several different eating-related difficulties. It is encountered in 30% to 50% of people with anorexia nervosa—that is, people who demonstrate an intense drive for thinness, self-imposed starvation, a refusal to maintain body weight at a level adequate for healthy functioning, and a belief that they are overweight despite emaciation. Binge eating is a significant problem also among the overweight. A series of studies assessing binge eating among people applying for behavioral weight-loss treatment reported rates between 23% and 46%. In a more recent study done at Stanford University, it was shown that the incidence of binge eating increases substantially with increasing levels of obesity. Binge eaters are more likely to drop out of weight-loss programs prematurely and to regain weight more quickly than nonbingers.

Binge eating is also one of the distinguishing characteristics of bulimia nervosa. Among people with this disorder, such episodes are usually followed by some form of purging, including self-induced vomiting or the use of laxatives. Some engage in vigorous exercise as a way of "undoing" the effects of a binge. Although the weight levels of people with bulimia nervosa are usually in the normal range, they are intensely preoccupied with their shape and have been described as "morbidly" frightened of becoming overweight. Binge eating and the associated methods of purging can cause serious medical problems, including menstrual disturbances, erosion of dental enamel and tooth loss, acute gastric dilation and rupture, esophageal rupture, and electrolyte imbalances that can lead to heart rhythm disturbances. Studies of the incidence of the "binge-purge syndrome" have indicated that it is almost exclusively confined to women and that as many as 15% of college-aged females may suffer such symptoms.

Among sufferers of bulimia nervosa, binges often alternate with attempts to rigidly restrict food intake. Elaborate "food rules" are common. One frequently encountered rule is to avoid eating sweets. Thus, if even one cookie or doughnut is consumed, the person may feel that she has "broken a rule" and must "get rid of" the objectionable food. Usually this leads to further overeating, both because it is easier to regurgitate a large amount of food than a small amount and because "having blown it," a decision is made to "go all the way" and start over tomorrow. In some cases, binges are triggered by negative mood states such as depression or anger.

COGNITIVE-BEHAVIORAL THERAPY

Most of the effort to develop effective psychologic treatment for binge eating has been directed toward bulimics who both binge and purge—that is, those with bulimia nervosa. Cognitive-behavioral therapy has been the most extensively evaluated therapy and appears at this point to be the most effective. This type of therapy focuses on helping patients alter beliefs and assumptions that are believed to be critical in maintaining bulimic behavior. The patient is asked to act as if she were a scientist testing assumptions and beliefs about food and weight as though they were hypotheses for conducting an experiment. The patient and therapist engage in a collaborative effort to examine the evidence regarding the validity of such beliefs. Usually, the evidence gathering and hypothesis testing involves the patient in a series of tests performed outside the therapy session. Among the procedures typical of cognitive-behavioral therapy for bulimia nervosa are the following.

Self monitoring of food intake and purging episodes. Patients are asked to keep detailed records indicating when they eat, what and how much they have consumed, whether they consider what they ate to be a binge, whether they purged, and the thoughts and feelings they had surrounding each episode of eating and purging. This procedure allows the patient and therapist jointly to examine patterns of thinking, feeling, and behavior that become the focus of efforts to change.

Normalization of the eating pattern. Patients are encouraged gradually to eat three adequate meals daily. This pattern breaks the binge-starve cycle that is so much a part of this problem. It also is a way of testing the validity of certain frequently reported beliefs among bulimics, such as "I will gain weight if I don't starve myself."

The addition of "forbidden foods" in small quantities to the diet. Rigid food rules are important in maintaining bulimia. If the person eats even a small amount of a forbidden food, it usually leads to a binge. Thus, one way that patients are encouraged to experiment with a less-rigid set of rules is to gradually add to their diets in smaller quantities foods that are forbidden.

Cognitive restructuring. The term *cognitive restructuring* refers to a set of procedures for identifying and attempting to correct "irrational" or maladaptive beliefs. All of the preceding tasks are designed to challenge such assumptions. However, cognitive-behavioral therapy for bulimia nervosa also involves direct identification and challenge of distortions in thinking that are associated with the disturbance. For example,

perfectionism and "all-or-nothing" thinking is common among this group. One is either eating correctly or horribly; one's weight is "acceptable" at 125 pounds and "totally unacceptable" at 126 pounds. Helping patients become aware of such thinking patterns and attempting to alter them is an important part of treatment. Patients are also encouraged to critically examine their attitudes toward body image, including what often amounts to rigid adherence to cultural stereotypes regarding thinness; they are also urged to reconsider the extent to which self-esteem is equated with body weight.

Identification of antecedents to binges and development of alternative coping strategies. One of the advantages of the self-monitoring procedure is that it enables the therapist and patient to identify events that seem to "trigger" binge episodes and allows the patient to explore alternative solutions for coping with those events. Sometimes, in addition to anxiety over a lapse in one's adherence to strict food rules, interpersonal situations may trigger binging; at other times negative emotional states such as depression, anxiety, or anger precipitate binges. Once such patterns are identified, alternative coping strategies can be developed, and the patient can begin to experiment with them.

HOW HELPFUL IS COGNITIVE-BEHAVIORAL TREATMENT?

Several published studies have indicated reductions in the incidence of binge eating and self-induced vomiting ranging from 63% to 96% after cognitive-behavioral therapy. The percentage of participants who abstain from binging and vomiting after such treatment has generally ranged between 50% and 60%. In the most recent study completed at Stanford University, cognitive-behavioral therapy resulted in a 77% reduction in purging; 59% of the participants were abstaining from binging and purging 6 months after treatment. In addition, participants showed significant improvement in other areas, such as depression and food preoccupation.

Although such results are most encouraging, it is obvious that not everyone benefits from such treatment. What can be said about those who do versus those who do not derive benefit? One factor that has been associated with poor outcome in cognitive-behavioral treatment for bulimia has been a history of anorexia. Excessive preoccupation with body shape and appearance is an important feature of bulimia nervosa, but it is possible that people with a history of anorexia are prone to *more* extreme preoccupation and are unable to tolerate the anxiety associated with experimenting with eating forbidden foods and developing a less-restrictive eating pattern. In a group of studies done at Stanford that have evaluated cognitive-behavioral therapy, weight gain has averaged only 2 pounds. Although we repeat this to most patients, some have difficulty being reassured, or find even 2 pounds intolerable.

In my experience, another major factor influencing success and failure is the patient's ability to enter into an open, collaborative relationship with the therapist. One characteristic of bulimic patients is preoccupation with the expectations of others. The therapy discussed here involves direct suggestions by the therapist. Although many patients welcome such focus and direction, some respond as though they are being evaluated on their ability to carry out the therapeutic tasks. Such patients are likely to feel that they have let the therapist down if they experience difficulty, or may expect that the therapist will become angry or punitive if improvement is not rapid enough. Others respond to the suggestions as though they are being coerced and "rebel" against what they perceive as the therapist's attempts to control their behavior. Cognitive-behavioral therapy is action-oriented; the cognitive change, or insight, that leads to therapeutic success derives not only from discussions with the therapist, but from actions carried out by the patient. To the extent that the patient is unable to collaborate with the therapist on the execution of those tasks, the therapy is undermined.

Although cognitive-behavioral therapy has been evaluated as a treatment for people with the binge-purge syndrome, it might prove to be an equally effective treatment for those who binge-eat without purging. Studies investigating its efficacy with that population are now being carried out.

Source: Bruce Arrow, *Healthline* (May 1990), pp. 2–4.

---

physiological abnormalities and emotional problems. These psychological deficits (low self-esteem, for example) contribute to the anorexic's apathy and unyielding stance in therapy. These problems are not nearly as prominent in treating bulimics.

Although forced vomiting is the most common means of purging to restrict calorie intake, other techniques are frequently used.

Laxative abuse is quite frequent as are **diuretic** and **emetic** abuse, fasting and enemas. The women are likely to exercise compulsively, swimming many laps, running many miles, working out with barbells and weights. Some women combine different methods of exercise as well as experimenting with bizarre diets. A small percentage of women we have treated spend hours chewing food and spitting it out. [11]

Diuretic: A drug designed to help the body convert excess water to urine; because they reduce the amount of water stored in the body, diuretic use often results in short-term weight loss and they are sometimes used for this purpose.

Emetic: A medication or substance used to induce vomiting.

The reasons for binging and purging are many and varied. Some of the more common ones are to avoid sexual relations, to

FIGURE 6.3
Bulimia

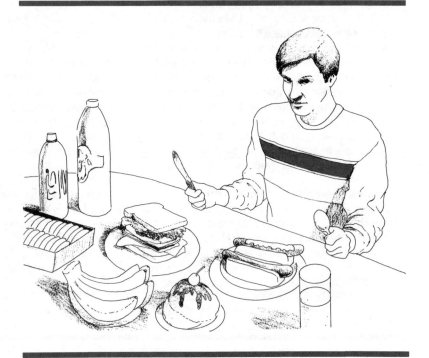

Bulimia is an eating disorder characterized by the consumption of enormous quantities of food followed by either forced vomiting or the abuse of laxatives or diuretics.

get attention, to get back at those people who "made her binge," to avoid the stress of new activities, and to avoid failure. In the case of those wanting to avoid failure, the binging and purging become the reason for all other failures. It is easier to blame failing a test, for example, on binging than to admit that the failure was the result of not studying. In addition to these reasons, socialization, the family, and the cults of slimness and youthfulness probably play major roles in bulimia.

Although a variety of treatment strategies has been tried with bulimics, there is still more we need to know. It would seem, however, that the outlook for bulimics of normal weight is better than for anorexics who binge and purge or for bulimics who abuse alcohol, other drugs, or whose condition is severe. For anorexics, the most common cause of death is **cachexia**, or wasting away. For bulimics, suicide is the most common cause of death. [12]

One recent and somewhat controversial method for treating bulimia involves the use of **antidepressant** drugs. Evidence is mounting that antidepressant drugs can quickly reduce binging and purging in some bulimics. Since it is believed that bulimic behavior often results directly from acute anxiety, low feelings of self-worth, or depression, antidepressants can help to counter these negative mood swings and reduce the incidence of negative behavior. There are, however, problems with this form of treatment that raise questions concerning its worth. First, antidepressants have a variety of side effects and can be fatal if overdosed. Bulimics often have suicidal tendencies, so putting such drugs in the hands of a bulimic is questionable. Second, studies have shown that when the drugs are discontinued, symptoms of bulimia return at disturbingly high rates. While antidepressant treatment may hide the symptoms, it does little or nothing to solve the underlying problems causing bulimia. [13] At best these drugs should be used on a short-term basis in conjunction with therapy.

HELP WITH EATING DISORDERS

With the recent public awareness of anorexia and bulimia, much attention has been focused on available treatments. Many private nutritional counselors and therapists have extended their practices to include the treatment of anorexia and bulimia, as have psychiatrists and psychological counselors. Overeaters Anonymous has helped some victims, while women's consciousness-raising groups and assertiveness-training groups have aided others. Self-help or social support groups have also proven valuable in treating sufferers. These groups are often led by women who have overcome anorexia or bulimia in the past. Their insights into the problems associated with these disorders can be most helpful. For more information on anorexia and bulimia, contact appropriate community resources. Some of these organizations are listed in the resource appendix in the back of this book.

A PLAN FOR ACTION

As with all areas of health, working on your weight or body composition requires effective decision-making. Remember to:

Cachexia: Massive weight loss, emaciation, and ill health caused by starvation.

Antidepressant: A class of durgs used to treat depression; antidepressants affect mood by raising the level of certain chemicals manufactured by the brain (neurotransmitters) that stimulate brain cell activity.

1. Identify the problem.

2. Identify all possible alternatives.

3. Look at the pros and cons of each alternative.

4. Select one alternative to try.

5. Evaluate and, if necessary, revise the alternative selected.

The first decision to be made is whether you really need to lose weight, and, if so, how much. This can best be accomplished by obtaining some type of body composition analysis. You should choose the most accurate method available. If no better methods are available, use your Body Mass Index as described in chapter 1. Once you know your percentage of body fat, decide what level of fat is desirable and feasible to obtain. You should make this decision with the help and guidance of a nutrition or weight-control counselor or a personal physician. Once you have determined your body composition and set appropriate goals, you should choose a good method. Since the most effective way to lose weight is to combine diet, exercise, and behavior modification, you should make decisions regarding each of these. Diet may be the most difficult thing to determine because such a wide variety of diets, diet advice, and diet products is available.

Choose an exercise program carefully as well. Your selections should be based on your goals (e.g., burning calories, increasing lean muscle mass, cardiovascular conditioning, and so on), current level of fitness, availability of time, and cost. Poor activity selection can result in physical injury or frustration, boredom, and, eventually, dropping the exercise program.

Finally, if the program is to be successful and long-lasting, you must decide to change your life-style. Going back to previous eating and exercise patterns will cause your body fat to return or increase. Behavior-modification strategies can help implement the initial life-style changes necessary to reduce body fat percentage and help maintain those changes once you have achieved a desirable body composition. Only you can make the proper decisions regarding which behaviors to modify and how best to do so. If you need further information to make a good decision, consult self-help books, weight-control counselors, and weight-control support groups.

Many people are concerned about their percentage of body fat and want to do something about it. Unfortunately, the vast majority are either unwilling or unable to accomplish this successfully. If you are serious about altering your body composition, however, here's some helpful advice:

1. Have a body composition analysis done. This is necessary to make sound decisions regarding the amount of weight (if any) to be lost. In addition, a body composition analysis may help motivate you to get started and, once you have begun, to stick with the program.

2. Select a well-balanced diet that contains a wide variety of foods to choose from and that takes a conservative approach to weight control. Try the diet for several weeks. If its requirements prove difficult to meet, make the necessary modifications.

3. Select an appropriate exercise program, one that can play an equal role with the diet selected as part of the total weight-control program. Schedule specific times to exercise daily. Stick to those times. If possible, find an exercise partner for added motivation. Above all, start slowly and make the exercise period enjoyable. An unpleasant exercise program is difficult to stay with.

4. Study current eating patterns and decide which eating behaviors require modification. In addition, reevaluate techniques for purchasing, preparing, serving, and storing food. Use behavior-modification strategies to help with each of these changes.

5. If necessary, locate a support group to help you make lifestyle changes. Weight Watchers is one such program, but there are others that can provide similar services. Consult chapter 4 for assistance.

6. Set a realistic goal before beginning a weight-loss program. When you realize that goal, sufficient quantities of food should be added back to the diet so the desired body composition can be maintained. Be aware that anorexia and bulimia are serious problems; if you continue to lose weight after you have met your original goal, you should consider seeking assistance to help you stay on the right track. W

Glossary

A

Adipose tissue: Fat tissue.

Adipsin: An enzyme, produced by fat cells and circulated by the blood, that is thought to influence the body's appetite control and energy expenditure.

Amphetamine: A class of drugs that stimulate the nervous system, particularly those that promote the release of chemicals manufactured by the brain (neurotransmitters) that stimulate wakefulness; amphetamines, which are usually available only by prescription, also suppress the appetite and are a common ingredient in many over-the-counter diet aids.

Anorexia nervosa: An eating disorder characterized by chronic undereating or refusal to eat that results in severe weight loss and is prompted by an obsessive fear of becoming fat.

Antidepressant: A class of drugs used to treat depression; antidepressants affect mood by raising the level of certain chemicals manufactured by the brain (neurotransmitters) that stimulate brain cell activity.

Atherosclerosis: A buildup of cholesterol, fat, and cellular debris within the inner layer of the arteries.

B

Behavior: An observable action or response.

Behavior modification: To alter one's behavior intentionally, eliminating unwanted behaviors, through a process of evaluating existing behaviors, identifying those to be changed, implementing changed behavior, and monitoring the results.

Body composition: A breakdown of total body weight into the proportions or amounts attributable to the various components of the body, particularly the 3 major constituents: fat, muscle, and bone.

Body Mass Index: A method of establishing normal weight, grade 1 obesity, or grade 2 obesity through a mathematical formula, using one's weight and height as variables.

Bradycardia: An abnormally low heart rate (less than 60 beats per minute in an adult); bradycardia may or may not be an indicator of an underlying disorder.

Bulimia: An eating disorder characterized by ingesting large amounts of food over a short period of time, followed by forced vomiting to avoid weight gain.

C

Cachexia: Massive weight loss, emaciation, and ill health caused by starvation.

Caloric balance: When one's caloric intake is equal to the number of calories one expends in maintaining normal functioning plus daily activities and/or exercising.

Calorie: The most widely used measure of the energy content of foods, the term calorie is actually an abbreviated version of the more technically correct term, kilocalorie or kcal, defined as the amount of heat necessary to raise the temperature of one *kilogram* of water one degree Celsius at normal atmospheric pressure; sometimes confused with the "small calorie" used in physics and chemistry; the latter equals the amount of heat necessary to raise the temperature of one *gram* of water by one degree Celsius at normal atmospheric pressure.

Cellulite: Popular name for lumpy, dimpled fat deposits, particularly those sometimes found on the thighs and buttocks; experts agree that there is no difference between "cellulite" and other fatty deposits.

Cholesterol: A group of related white, waxy substances that are important components of the cell membranes in the body; several types of cholesterol are found in the blood including high density lipoproteins (HDL)—the so-called "good cholesterol" that seems to protect against arterial disease—and low density lipoprotiens (LDL) that seem to contribute to it and are thus sometimes known as "bad cholesterol."

Complex carbohydrate: A polysaccharide, or compound consisting of many sugar molecules linked together. Complex carbohydrates in the diet include starches and the fiber, cellulose.

Contracting: The practice of drawing up an agreement (usually written) between 2 or more persons for the purpose of assigning responsibility for carrying out a particular task or activity and establishing the conditions under which this is to occur.

D

Diabetes: A disorder characterized by abnormally high levels of glucose (sugar) in the blood resulting from the failure of the pancreas to produce a sufficient supply of insulin, the hormone responsible for the conversion of glucose into a form usable by the cells of the body; the major symptoms of diabetes are fatigue, weight loss, excessive urination, and thirst.

Diet: A person's ordinary and customary daily consumption of food and drink.

Dietary amenorrhea: The absence of menstruation resulting from severe weight loss.

Diet-help industry: The industry comprised of those firms and other organizations that produce and market programs, diet aids, and other materials or services designed to promote weight loss.

Diuretic: A drug designed to help the body convert excess water to urine; because they reduce the amount of water stored in the body, diuretic use often results in short-term weight loss and they are sometimes used for this purpose.

E

Eating disorder: A chronic pattern of abnormal dieting behavior that has negative health effects; the 2 best known eating disorders are anorexia nervosa and bulimia.

Eclampsia: A condition characterized by a series of seizures during late pregnancy, labor, or the postnatal period; can cause coma or death.

Electrical impedance: A method of determining amount of body fat by measuring the body tissue's resistance to a low-voltage electrical current. This method works on the principle that lean tissue and fat tissue conduct electricity differently.

Emetic: A medication or substance used to induce vomiting.

Empty foods: Foods that contain a high number of calories but provide little or no nutritional benefit; alcoholic beverages are often cited as an example of empty foods; see also junk food.

Endoscope: A lighted viewing instrument that can be inserted into a body cavity from the outside allowing visual examination of the interior of the body.

Essential fat: One of two major forms of body fat. Essential fat cells maintain normal physiological functioning and are found in bone marrow, the heart, lungs, spleen, kidneys, intestines, muscles, and nervous system.

F

Fad diets: Weight-loss eating programs taken up and followed with exaggerated zeal for a short time.

Fat cell theory: A hypothesis suggesting that the body increases the quantity of fat tissue in two ways: hypertrophy and/or hyperplasia.

Fat substitute: A food product designed to simulate the taste and texture of animal or vegetable fat while containing fewer calories.

Fat weight: The portion of total body weight attributed to fatty tissues.

G

Glucose: A monosaccharide or simple sugar found in foods by itself and also as part of complex carbohydrates and the disaccharides sucrose, maltose, and lactose; also known as blood sugar.

Glycogen: A form of complex carbohydrate stored in the body. It is found primarily in liver and muscle tissue.

H

Hyperplasia: One of two ways fat cell theory suggests that the body increases its fat tissue, by increasing the number of fat cells in the body.

Hypertension: Abnormally high blood pressure.

Hypertrophy: One of two ways fat cell theory suggests that the body increases its fat tissue, by enlarging fat cells that already exist in the body.

Hypotension: The medical term for abnormally low blood pressure.

Hypothalamus: A region of the brain located immediately below the thalamus and behind the eyes which regulates the portion of the nervous system that controls the internal organs of the body; the hypothalamus plays a major role in the regulation of body temperature, the so-called "fight or flight" response, and a broad range of other important functions.

I

Intestinal bypass surgery: A surgical procedure in which a portion of the small intestine is removed and the two ends rejoined thus shortening the overall length of the intestine; while formerly used as a treatment for obesity, this procedure is today most often employed in cancer patients.

Isometric exercise: An exercise in which a muscle or set of muscles is pitted against either an immovable object or another muscle or set of muscles.

J

Junk food: A popular term used to describe food that contains a high number of calories but is low in nutritional value, especially highly processed snack foods containing large amounts of refined sugar.

K

Ketogenic: Any behavior or activity that can cause ketosis, a potentially serious condition characterized by the accumulation of excessive amounts of ketone in the body. The symptoms of ketosis include irritability, weakness, and nausea.

Kilocalorie (kcal): The most widely used measure of the energy content of foods, a kilocalorie is defined as the amount of heat necessary to raise the temperature of one *kilogram* of water one degree Celsius at normal atmospheric pressure; commonly referred to as "calorie" and thus sometimes confused with the "small calorie" used in physics and chemistry; the latter equals the amount of heat necessary to raise the temperature of one *gram* of water by one degree Celsius at normal atmospheric pressure.

L

Lean body weight: That portion of total body weight that remains after subtracting fat weight, the portion of total body weight attributed to fatty tissues.

Life expectancy: The average number of years remaining in the life of a living being, it can be predicted at any time in the life of the being by averaging the age at death of all members of the species over a fixed period of time.

Life-style: A style of living that consistently reflects a particular set of values and attitudes.

Lipid: A class of fatty substances that are insoluble in water, transported throughout the body by the blood, and are one of the body's important sources of food energy; the more important types of lipids include triglycerides (the principal component of body fat) and sterols such as cholesterol.

Lipoprotein: A class of proteins found in the blood that consist of a simple protein combined with a lipid, a class of fatty substances that are insoluble in water, transported throughout the body by the blood, and are one of the body's important sources of food energy.

Liposuction: A surgical technique in which excess adipose tissue (storage fat) beneath the skin is removed by a suction device; also known as suction lipectomy.

M

Metabolic rate: A term used to describe the body's rate of metabolism, a general term for all of the chemical and physical processes that take place continuously within the living body.

Metabolism: The physical and chemical process whereby the body transforms food into energy by breaking large molecules into smaller molecules.

Mind-set: An established attitude or inclination toward a subject or situation.

N

Nutrient: A nourishing component of food that serves to sustain life, promote growth, prevent decay, or provide energy.

O

Obesity: The excessive accumulation of fat in the body to a level that, depending on the age, frame size, and height of the affected person, is considered undesirable.

Osteoarthritis: A common joint disease among elderly people, resulting from excessive wear on joints, sometimes due to obesity, slight deformity, or misalignment of bones. Common symptoms include pain, swelling, stiffness, joint distortion and enlargement, and weakness of surrounding muscles.

Overfat: Obese, indicating the excessive accumulation of fat in the body.

Over-the-counter (OTC) diet aid: Any of the variety of products that are promoted as helpful in losing weight and may be purchased without a prescription.

Overweight: A condition characterized by weight that exceeds what is considered normal and healthy, based on an average taken from people of comparable age, height, frame size, and sex.

P

Phenylpropanolamine (PPA): An appetite suppressant used to treat obesity. Prolonged use of this drug can lead to addiction, high blood pressure, nausea, and anxiety.

Plasma lipid: Any of the fatty, organic substances carried in the blood plasma, the fluid portion of the blood that remains after the blood cells have been removed.

Preeclampsia: A condition of late pregnancy; characterized by high blood pressure, fluid retention, and protein in the urine. If untreated, preeclampsia may lead to eclampsia.

R

Refined sugar: Term used to describe sweeteners such as white sugar that are created by processing and thus can be distinguished from natural sugars such as honey.

S

Satiety: The feeling of fullness that follows eating.

Self-efficacy: A belief in one's ability to control events or to accomplish one's objectives; a sense of self-confidence.

Setpoint theory: The hypothesis that the body has an internal control mechanism, centered in the brain, which strives to maintain the individual's predetermined body fat level.

Skinfold measurement: A method of determining the percentage of body fat by measuring folds of skin from several areas of the body with a specialized caliper.

Spa: An often luxurious, residential, resort-like facility that is operated on a commercial basis and offers a variety of health-related services including weight-reduction programs.

Spot reduction: The unfounded belief that exercising selected areas of the body will result in a greater loss of excess fat in that area than would otherwise occur as a result of whole-body exercise.

Storage fat: One of two major types of body fat. Storage fat cells accumulate as adipose tissue.

Subcutaneous: Beneath the skin, as in a subcutaneous injection.

Subcutaneous fat: A layer of fat found below the skin but over the muscles.

U

Underwater weighing: A method of determining amount of body fat using the principle that lean body tissue is denser than fat body tissue. While immersed in water, the lean, denser tissue will displace more water and weigh more than the fat, less dense tissue.

Underweight: A statistical designation based on total body weight which is 10 percent or more under the ideal weight indicated on a standard height and weight chart.

V

Very-low-calorie diet (VLCD): A medically supervised diet wherein the patient fasts for up to 12 weeks on food consisting of a powder formula mixed with water that provides essential nutrients while supplying only 400 to 600 calories per day.

W

Weight-loss diet: A plan of food and drink consumption followed in order to meet a specific weight-loss goal.

Y

Yo-yo effect: Rapid up-down-up weight fluctuations, a phenomenon common among dieters.

CHAPTER 1

1. F. I. Katch and W. D. McArdle, *Nutrition, Weight Control, and Exercise* 3d ed. (Philadelphia: Lea & Febiger, 1988), 137.
2. G. Kolata, "Why do people get fat?" *Science* (15 March 1985): 1327–1328.
3. National Institutes of Health Consensus Development Panel, "Health Implications of Obesity," *Annals of Internal Medicine* 103 (1985): 1073–1077.
4. "Prevalence of Overweight in Selected States–Behavioral Risk Factor Surveillance, 1986," *Journal of the American Medical Association* 259, no. 6 (1988): 796–798.
5. W. E. Leary, "Young Women Are Getting Fatter, Study Finds," *New York Times,* 23 February 1989, B10.
6. J. Carey and R. Taylor, "Battling the Bulge at an Early Age," *U.S. News and World Report,* 2 March 1987, 66–67.
7. Department of Health and Human Services, Public Health Service, *Promoting Health/Preventing Disease: Public Health Service Implementation Plans for Attaining the Objectives for the Nation* (Washington, DC: Government Printing Office, 1983).
8. E. Jequier, "Obesity and Body Weight Standards," *American Journal of Clinical Nutrition* 45 (1987): 1035–1047.
9. S. Fujioka et al., "Contribution of Intra-abdominal Fat Accumulation to the Impairment of Glucose and Lipid Metabolism in Human Obesity," *Metabolism* 36, no. 1 (January 1987): 54–59.
10. B. A. Brehm, "Abdominal Fat and Heart Disease Risk," *Fitness Management* 6, no. 12 (November 1990): 31–33.
11. Katch and McArdle, p. 137.
12. National Institutes of Health Consensus Development Panel, pp. 1073–1077.
13. P. A. Hillard, "Obesity in Pregnancy," *Parents,* December 1988, 200, 202.
14. Katch and McArdle, p. 137.
15. L. Baum, "Extra Pounds Can Weigh Down Your Career," *Business Week,* 3 August 1987, 96.
16. National Institutes of Health Consensus Development Panel, pp. 1073-1077.
17. See S. Orbach, *Fat is a Feminist Issue* (New York: Paddington Press, 1978), and K. Chernin, *The Obsession: Reflections on the Tyranny of Slenderness* (New York: Harper & Row, 1981).
18. Orbach, pp. 25–26.

CHAPTER 2

1. J. Hirsch and R. L. Leibel, "New Light on Obesity," *New England Journal of Medicine* 318, no. 8 (1988): 509–510.
2. T. J. Coates and C. C. Thoresen, "Treating Obesity in Adolescents and Children, A Review," *American Journal of Public Health* 68, no. 2 (1978): 145.
3. "Tipping the Scale," *Scientific American,* June 1986, 70.
4. C. Bouchard et al., "The Response to Long-Term Overfeeding in Identical Twins," *New England Journal of Medicine* 322, no. 21 (24 May 1990): 1477–1482.
5. A. J. Stunkard and B. Lawren, "Family Fat," *Health,* February 1987, 8.
6. Hirsch and Leibel, pp. 509–510.
7. G. Kolata, "Study Links Crash Dieting to Slower Weight Loss," *New York Times,* 1 July 1988, B6.
8. L. Bellini-Gergley, "Is Your Metabolism Too Slow?" *Mademoiselle,* August 1988, 142.
9. Katch and McArdle, p. 137.
10. J. S. Flier et al., "Severly Impaired Adipsin Expression in Genetic and Acquired Obesity," *Science* 237 (1987): 405–408.
11. Flier et al., pp. 405–408.
12. A. S. Moffat, "Genetics or Gluttony," *American Health* (September 1988): 106.
13. Katch and McArdle, p. 137.
14. Roberts et al., "Energy Expenditure and Intake in Infants Born to Lean and Overweight Mothers," *New England Journal of Medicine* 318, no. 8 (25 February 1988): 461–466.
15. J. Mayer, "Hidden Bonds," *World Health* (February/March 1974): 21–27.
16. B. Q. Haffen, *Nutrition, Food and Weight Control* (Boston: Allyn and Bacon, 1981).

CHAPTER 3

1. Katch and McArdle, 1988, and Brownell, "Exercise and Obesity," *Behavioral Medicine Update* 4, no. 1 (1982), 7–11.
2. Katch and McArdle, p. 175.
3. Katch and McArdle, p. 175.
4. F. I. Katch et al., "Preferential Effects of Abdominal Exercise Training on Regional Adipose Cell Size," *Research Quarterly for Exercise and Sport* 55 (1984): 249.
5. Katch et al., pp. 150–151.
6. "Walking Your Way."

7. J. H. Wilmore and D. L. Costill, *Training for Sport and Activity* (Dubuque, IA: Wm. C. Brown, 1988).
8. Wilmore and Costill.
9. Wilmore and Costill.

CHAPTER 4

1. P. Long, "Fat Chance," *Hippocrates* (September/October 1989): 39–47.
2. "Weight Control: New Findings," *Dairy Council Digest* 55, no. 3 (May/June 1988): 13–18.
3. P. McCarthy, "The Waist Wars: Fighting in the Aisles," *Psychology Today*, November 1986, 8–10.
4. L. E. Grahm III et al., "Five Year Follow-up to a Behavioral Weight Loss Program," *Journal of Consulting and Clinical Psychology* 51, no. 2 (1983): 322–323.
5. K. J. Hartigan, P. Baker-Strauch, and G. W. Moris, "Perceptions of the Causes of Obesity and Responsiveness to Treatment," *Journal of Consulting Psychology* 29, no. 5 (1982): 478–485.
6. R. O. Nelson, "Assessment and Therapeutic Functions of Self-monitoring," in *Progress in Behavior Modification* vol. 5, M. Hersen, R. M. Eisler, and P. M. Miller, eds. (New York: Academic Press, 1977).
7. R. Cameron and J. A. Best, "Promoting Adherence to Health Behavior Change Interventions: Recent Findings From Behavioral Research," *Patient Education and Counseling* 10 (1987): 139–154.
8. E. A. Locke et al., "Goal Setting and Task Performance: 1969–1980," *Psychological Bulletin* 90 (1981): 125–152.
9. Cameron and Best, pp. 139–154.
10. Cameron and Best, pp. 139–154.
11. Nelson.
12. Locke et al., pp. 125–152.
13. G. Ainslie, "Rationality and the Emotions: A Picoeconomic Approach," *Social Science Information* 24, no. 2 (1985): 355–374.
14. M. R. Lepper, D. Greene, and R. E. Nisbett, "Undermining Children's Intrinsic Interest with Extrinsic Rewards: A Test of the 'Overjustification' Hypotheses," *Journal of Personal and Social Psychology* 28 (1973): 129–137.
15. K. E. Grady, C. Goodenow, and J. R. Borkin, "The Effect of Reward on Compliance with Breast Self-Examination," *Journal of Behavioral Medicine* 11, vol. 1 (1988): 43–57.

16. Grady, Goodenow, and Borkin, pp. 43–57.

17. Cameron and Best, pp. 139–154, and S. P. Singleton et al., "Behavioral Contracting in an Urban Health Promotion Project," *Evaluation and the Health Professions* 10, vol. 4 (1987): 408–437.

18. K. Lewin, *Field Theory in Social Science: Selected Theoretical Papers* (Chicago: The University of Chicago Press, 1951), 9–18, 23.

19. N. Henderson, "Crying the Weight-Loss Blues," *Changing Times,* April 1989, 75–78.

20. B. O'Reilly, "Diet Centers are Really in Fat City," *Fortune,* 5 June 1989, 137–140.

21. L. R. Franzini and W. B. Grimes, "Treatment Strategies for Therapists Conducting Weight Control Programs," *Psychotherapy: Theory, Research and Practice* 181 (1981): 81–93, and W. A. Sperduto and R. M. O'Brien, "Effects of Cash Deposits on Attendance and Weight Loss in a Large Scale Clinical Program for Obesity," *Psychological Reports* 52, vol. 1 (1983): 261–262.

22. R. W. Jeffery et al., "Monetary Contracts in Weight Control: Effectiveness of Group and Individual Contracts of Varying Size," *Journal of Consulting and Clinical Psychology* 51, vol. 2 (1983): 242–248.

CHAPTER 5

1. M. A. Webster, *Webster's New Collegiate Dictionary* (Springfield, MA: G. & C. Merriam, 1979), 407.

2. S. R. Morrow and L. K. Mona, "Effect of Gastric Balloons on Nutrient Intake and Weight Loss in Obese Subjects," *Journal of the American Dietetic Association* 90, vol. 5 (May 1990): 717–718.

3. G. A. Bray, "Obesity: A Blueprint for Progress," *Contemporary Nutrition* 12, no. 7 (1987), and "Bubble Trouble," *HMS Health Letter* (August 1987): 3–4.

4. "Position of The American Dietetic Association: Very-Low Calorie Weight Loss Diets," *Journal of the American Dietetic Association* 90, vol. 5 (May 1990): 722–726.

5. "Position of the American Dietetic Association," pp. 722–726.

6. L. Zinn, "Sipping Your Way into Slimmer Shape," *Business Week,* 31 October 1988, 162–163, and A. Sachs, "Drinking Yourself Skinny," *Time,* 19 December 1988, 68.

7. J. E. Brody, "Diet that Made Oprah Winfrey Slim Demands

Discipline, Specialists Say," *New York Times*, 24 November 1988, B17.

8. "Not So Simplesse," *University of California, Berkeley Wellness Letter* 6, vol. 10 (July 1990): 2.

9. "Getting the Fat Out to Make Food Healthier," *Calorie Control Commentary* 12, vol. 2 (Fall 1990): 1–6.

10. "Paring Off Pounds at a Live-in Clinic," *Changing Times*, February 1986, 71–74.

CHAPTER 6

1. A. Drewnowski, S. A. Hopkins, and R. C. Kessler, "The Prevalence of Bulimia Nervosa in the U.S. College Student Population," *American Journal of Public Health* 78, no. 10 (October 1988): 1322–1324.

2. F. Litsky, "Neyer Wins a Personal Battle," *New York Times*, 30 November 1988, C3.

3. J. E. Brody, "The Resurgence of Anorexia, the Emotional Disease of Young Women Bent on Starvation," *New York Times HEALTH*, 19 May 1988, B14.

4. J. H. Swarth, "Relationship Between Food Attitudes and Dietary Practices of College Women" (Unpublished Masters Thesis: University of Oregon, 1984).

5. D. E. Schotte and A. J. Stunkard, "Bulimia vs. Bulimic Behaviors on a College Campus," *Journal of the American Medical Association* 258, no. 9 (4 September 1987): 1213–1215.

6. "Eating Disorders," *Dairy Council Digest* 56, no. 1 (1985): 1.

7. P. E. Garfunkel and D. M. Garner, *Anorexia Nervosa: A Multidimensional Perspective* (New York: Bruner Mazel Publications, 1982).

8. "Eating Disorders," p. 1.

9. A. Drewnowski et al., pp. 1322–1324.

10. "Eating Disorders," p. 1.

11. M. Boskind-White and W. C. White, *Bulimarexia: The Binge/Purge Cycle* (New York: W. W. Norton and Co., 1983), 44.

12. "Eating Disorders," p. 1.

13. "Drugs Win Support as a Bulimia Treatment," *New York Times*, 22 March 1988, C7.

BOOKS

Bailey, Covert. *Fit or Fat Target Diet.* Boston: Houghton Mifflin, 1984.

This book is easy to read, humorous, and makes important points about exercise and diet. It works well as a beginner's book to help get readers interested in exercise and to help them realize that dieting alone cannot help in controlling weight. The author maintains that all the vitamins and minerals that the average healthy person needs can be obtained by eating the right foods, without need for supplements. Bailey's target diet focuses on eating a balanced diet from all the major food groups and eating foods low in fat, low in sugar, and high in fiber.

Brody, Jane. *Jane Brody's Nutrition Book.* New York: Bantam Books, 1987.

A comprehensive guide by the *New York Times*'s health journalist, covering nutrients, nutrition guidelines, nutrition and disease, weight management, food labeling, and the special needs of athletes, pregnant women, children, adolescents, the elderly, and vegetarians. The author explains the "whys" behind good eating and the "hows" of making sensible dietary changes.

Brody, Jane. *The New York Times Guide to Personal Health.* New York: The New York Times Book Co., 1982.

Based on Jane Brody's award-winning and immensely popular "Personal Health" columns from the *New York Times,* this book tells you how to take charge of your health. It shows you how to stay healthy, how to participate in your medical care, what to do when things go wrong, how to avoid unnecessary and expensive treatment, and how to get better care from your doctors. The goal of the text is to maximize your chances for a healthy and active old age while making the most of all the years of your life. It is both a lifetime guide to healthful living and a handy medical companion to help you deal with everyday panics and problems. The fifteen sections cover nutrition, exercise, emotional health, environmental health effects, common serious illnesses, and more.

Burstein, Nancy. *Soft Aerobics: The New Low-Impact Workout.* New York: G. P. Putnam, 1987.

This book presents an alternative to traditional, high-impact aerobics which can cause injury from excess stress on ankles, shins, calves, knees, hips, and back. Twelve low-impact exercises combined into 4 different exercise routines are presented. Illustrated with step-by-step photographs so you can follow the specific routines presented in the book or create your own personalized program for your individual fitness level.

Connor, Sonja L., M.S., and William E. Connor, M.D. *The New American Diet: The Lifetime Family Eating Plan for Good Health.* New York: Simon & Schuster, 1986.

A lifetime eating guide for families that emphasizes gradual change into healthier eating habits, particularly lower fat intake. The diet is divided into three phases. Phase One is the modification of present recipes and eating habits. Phase Two begins to lower meat consumption and present new recipes. Phase Three incorporates beans and grains as the main protein sources, without the fat.

Cooper, Kenneth H. *Controlling Cholesterol: Dr. Kenneth H. Cooper's Preventive Medicine Program.* New York: Bantam, 1988.

The author presents a program for identifying and reducing your risk of heart disease and for controlling your cholesterol level. Also discussed are diet, alcohol, smoking, exercise, stress, birth control pills, fish oil, fiber, how to obtain an accurate blood-cholesterol profile, and other topics.

Edwards, Ted L., with Barbara Lau. *Weight Loss to Super Wellness.* 2d ed. Austin, TX: Hills Medical/Sports, 1988.

Edwards, a weight-loss lecturer and expert in preventive medicine, presents a diet rich in fiber and an exercise program to fit anyone's life-style. He explains why fad diets fail, how these crash diets can actually result in weight gain, how to control food cravings, and how mental attitudes can affect health and wellness. The author also presents advice on ending the need for tobacco and how massage and biofeedback can induce relaxation and lead to greater health.

Eisenman, Patricia A., Stephen C. Johnson, and Joan E. Benson. *Coaches' Guide to Nutrition and Weight Control.* 2d ed. Champaign, IL: Human Kinetics Publishers, 1989.

A popular and practical guide about sport nutrition and how to present this information to athletes. Complete nutrition information is given, including information on amino acid supplements and eating disorders. Information from the sciences of physiology, biochemistry, and nutrition are brought together and presented clearly by the authors and can be applied easily to any sport. This book is part of the ACEP Master Series Sport Science Curriculum.

Ferguson, James M., M.D. *Habits, Not Diets: The Secret to Lifetime Weight Control.* Palo Alto, CA: Bull Publishing, 1988.

A fine handbook that focuses on behavior change and eating patterns for permanent weight management. Emphasizes an active life-style, stress management, behavior change skills, and how to eat rather than what to eat. Also covers stress management and includes instructions and forms for a self-directed weight management program.

Fletcher, Anne M. *Eat Fish, Live Better.* New York: Harper & Row, 1989.

In this book the author explains how to buy, store, clean, and cook fish, and why fish should be added to your diet to aid in the prevention of heart disease. Based on medical and scientific findings, the book shows that a greater fish intake leads to lower fat consumption and greater health. Includes 75 fat-reducing recipes.

Franks, B. Don, and Edward T. Howley. *Fitness Facts: The Healthy Living Handbook.* Champaign, IL: Human Kinetics Publishers, 1989.

Discussed in this book are how to test one's fitness, improve one's fitness level, and set up an individual fitness program based on current research. The authors answer many basic questions about exercise and fitness. Chapters present fitness progress self-evaluation questions, definitions of fitness, how to change to more healthful behaviors, selecting the right fitness program, injury prevention, and more.

Guide to More Healthful Living. Edited by the Blue Cross/Blue Shield Association. New York: Contemporary Books, 1986.

A complete guide to maintaining overall wellness of body and mind. Written and compiled by nine medical doctors, chapter titles include "Wellness," "Nutrition," "Physical Fitness," "Reducing Stress," and "Your Health and Fitness Life-style." Two additional sections include

"Your Health Best Score Card," which allows you to chart your health progress, and "The Life Management Self-Evaluation Test," which includes questions about eating habits, physical activity, environment, smoking habits, and stress evaluations. The book is designed so you can determine your own total life management score.

Jennings-Sauer, Cheryl. *Living Lean by Choosing More.* Virginia City, MT: O. J. Taylor, 1989.

This book emphasizes gradual life-style and eating habit changes to result in permanent weight loss through an eight-week program. Based on scientific research of metabolism and weight-loss psychology, this book is more than just another diet book.

Kingsbury, Bonnie D. *Full Figure Fitness: A Program for Teaching Overweight Adults.* Champaign, IL: Human Kinetics Publishers, 1988.

A quality exercise program for fitness instructors and exercise specialists to use with overweight adults. This book helps obese adults understand the complex nature of obesity and offers practical advice from experts in psychology, physical therapy, and nutrition. Kingsbury based this book on her many years of teaching fitness classes to overweight adults. Provided also is marketing and promotional information for fitness instructors to set up a Full Figure Fitness program. The book is useful to individuals who want to know more about appropriate exercise programs for the overweight adult.

Meyers, Casey. *Aerobic Walking: The Best and Safest Weight Loss and Cardiovascular Exercise for Everyone Overweight or Out of Shape.* New York: Random House, 1987.

This book addresses the benefits of walking for the purpose of disease prevention and helping with weight-control problems. Covered are the proper walking gait for maximum aerobic benefits and reduced stress on joints, and how to develop a self-tailored fitness walking program.

Nash, Joyce D. *Maximize Your Body Potential: Sixteen Weeks to a Lifetime of Effective Weight Management.* Palo Alto, CA: Bull Publishing, 1986.

The book includes personal weight-loss and exercise programs, how to change behavior and cope with life problems that impact on successful weight management. Works as a teaching text and as a personal weight-control program.

Popular Diets: How They Rate. 2d ed. Los Angeles: California Dietetic Association, 1987.

This book provides an analysis of 15 popular diets and 2 weight-loss programs. Each diet has a description, rationale, computer analysis (based on a 3-day sample menu), evaluation, and recommendation. The RDAs and the Dietary Guidelines for All Americans are two nutritional guidelines used for each analysis.

Robertson, Laurel, Carol Flinders, and Brian Ruppenthal. *The New Laurel's Kitchen.* 2d ed. Berkeley, CA: Ten Speed Press, 1986.

Almost every recipe from the original edition of this vegetarian book has been updated to lower fat content or enhance nutrition. Contains over 150 completely new recipes and extensive tables showing the nutrition composition of each food mentioned in the recipes. A good book for healthful cooking for vegetarians.

Tribole, Evelyn, M.S., R.D. *Eating on the Run.* Champaign, IL: Life Enhancement Publications, 1987.

A helpful handbook that shows how to work a balanced diet into a busy schedule. Includes guidelines for choices in fast-food restaurants, selecting frozen convenience foods, and preparing quick meals in 60 seconds or less. The author also provides weight-control techniques, meal and snack planning strategies, 24 quick recipes, and caloric and nutrition content charts.

NEWSLETTERS

ASCH News and Views is published five times a year by the American Council on Science and Health, a nonprofit educational association promoting scientifically balanced evaluations of food, chemicals, the environment, and health. A one-year subscription is $15. Write to ASCH News and Views, 1995 Broadway, New York, NY 10023, or call (212) 362-7044.

Consumer Reports Health Letter is published monthly by Consumers Union of the United States, a nonprofit organization that provides information and advice on goods, services, health, and personal finance. A one-year subscription is $24, and two years cost $38. Write to the Subscription Director, Consumer Reports Health Letter, Box 56356, Boulder, CO 80322-6356, or call (800) 274-8370.

Environmental Nutrition: The Professional Newsletter of Diet, Nutrition, and Health is an interesting monthly publication featuring informative and reliable articles on diet and nutrition. A one-year subscription is $36. Write to Environmental Nutrition, 2112 Broadway, New York, NY 10023.

Harvard Health Letter is published monthly as a nonprofit service by the Department of Continuing Education, Harvard Medical School, in association with Harvard University Press. The letter has the goal of interpreting health information for general readers in a timely and accurate fashion. A one-year subscription is $21. Write to the Harvard Medical School Letter, 79 Garden Street, Cambridge, MA 02138, or call customer service at (617) 495-3975.

Healthline is published monthly by Healthline Publishing, Inc. The letter is intended to educate readers about ways to help themselves avoid illness and live longer, healthier lives. A one-year subscription is $19, or $34 for two years. Write to Healthline, The C. V. Mosby Company, 11830 Westline Industrial Drive, St. Louis, MO 63146-3318, or call (800) 325-4177 (ext. 351).

Johns Hopkins Medical Letter, Health After 50 is published monthly by Medletter Associates, Inc., and covers a variety of topics related to healthful living. A one-year subscription is $20. Write to the Johns Hopkins Medical Letter, P.O. Box 420179, Palm Coast, FL 32142.

Mayo Clinic Nutrition Letter is published monthly and provides reliable information about nutrition and fitness and how decisions on these matters affect your health. A one-year subscription is $24. Write to the Mayo Foundation for Medical Education and Research, 200 1st Street SW, Rochester, MN 55905, or call (800) 888-3968.

Running & FitNews is published monthly by the American Running and Fitness Association, a nonprofit educational association of athletes and sports medicine professionals. This newsletter provides information on exercise guidelines, injuries, diet, and health-related fitness topics. A one-year subscription is $25. Write to the AR&FA, 9310 Old Georgetown Road, Bethesda, MD 20814, or call (301) 897-0197.

Tufts University Diet and Nutrition Letter is published monthly and covers topics related to health and wellness, including exercise, nutrition, environmental factors, smoking, and so on. A one-year subscription costs $20. Write to the Tufts

University Diet and Nutrition Letter, 53 Park Place, New York, NY 10007.

University of California Berkeley Wellness Letter is published monthly and covers many topics, including nutrition, fitness, and stress management. A one-year subscription is $20. Write to the University of California, Berkeley Wellness Letter, P.O. Box 420148, Palm Coast, FL 32142.

PERIODICALS

American Health Magazine: Fitness of Body and Mind is published 10 times a year and covers every aspect of physical and mental well-being. In addition to feature articles, ongoing departments include Nutrition News, Fitness Reports, Mind/Body News, Family Report, Family Pet, and more. A one-year subscription is $14.95. Write to American Health: Fitness of Body and Mind, P.O. Box 3015, Harlan, IA 51537-3015.

Cooking Light Magazine is published 6 times a year. Developed by nutritionists and dieticans, this colorful magazine provides a wealth of information on cooking with less fat and sugar and contains interesting food and nutrition articles, practical meal planning information, and creative recipes with amounts of fat, cholesterol, sodium, and calories per serving provided. A one-year subscription is $12. Write to Cooking Light, P.O. Box C-549, Birmingham, AL 35283.

Health Magazine is published 10 times a year by Family Media, Inc. This magazine also features a half-dozen articles per issue on fitness for both mind and body, environmental topics, sporting activities, health, and food. It has a regular Healthline section dealing with topics related to behavior, medical information, and children's health. A one-year subscription is $19.95. Write to Health Magazine, Subscription Dept., P.O. Box 420030, Palm Coast, FL 32142-0030, or call (800) 423-1780; in Florida (800) 858-0095.

In Health Magazine is published 6 times a year and provides articles on a number of health issues. In addition to recipes and practical nutrition tips, the magazine regularly includes self-help resources for consumers. A one-year subscription is $18. Write to In Health, P.O. Box 52431, Boulder, CO 80321-2431.

Priorities: For Long Life & Good Health is published quarterly by the American Council of Science and Health, Inc. (ACSH), a nonprofit consumer education association promoting scientifically balanced evaluations of nutrition, chemicals, life-style factors, the environment, and human health. General individual membership in ACSH, which includes a subscription to Priorities, costs $25 a year. Write to the Subscription Department, Priorities, 1995 Broadway, 16th Floor, New York, NY 10023-5860.

Saint Raphael's Better Health is published bimonthly by the Better Health Press, a division of the Institute for Better Health, in cooperation with the Hospital of Saint Raphael, New Haven, Connecticut. Both are nonprofit organizations, and the magazine is designed to further readers' understanding of how to maintain good health. A one-year subscription is free, but a modest, nonmandatory annual donation is requested to help defray publication costs. Write to Better Health, 1384 Chapel Street, New Haven, CT 06511, or call (203) 789-3972.

HOTLINES

American Diabetes Association, (800) ADA-DISC. Staff members will answer general questions about diabetes, risk factors, and symptoms. Free literature, and a free quarterly newsletter, *Diabetes '91*, will be sent upon request. Service available 8:30 A.M. to 5:00 P.M., Eastern Standard Time, Monday through Friday.

American Dietetic Association, (800) 877-1600. The American Dietetic Association (ADA) is the major professional organization for the dietetic profession. The ADA will answer questions and provide information to callers on subjects related to foods and nutrition.

National Health Information Center, Department of Health and Human Services,(800) 336-4797. Operated by the Office of Disease Prevention and Health Promotion, this information and referral center's trained personnel will direct you to the organization or government agency that can assist you with your health question, whether it's about high blood pressure, cancer, fitness, or any other topic. Available 9:00 A.M. to 5:00 P.M., Eastern Standard Time, Monday through Friday.

Tel-Med is a free telephone service provided in many cities. You can call and ask for a specific tape number, and have the health message played for you over the phone. There are over 300 medical topics to choose from, including topics related to maintaining a healthy life-style, and many states provide toll-free numbers for this service. Call your local information operator to find the nearest Tel-Med office, or write to Tel-Med, Box 970, Colton, CA 92324.

VIDEOTAPES

The following video programs related to wellness and weight-control topics can be ordered from the National Wellness Institute, Inc., South Hall, 1319 Fremont Street, Stevens Point, WI 54481. Write for format, price, and ordering information.

Living With High Blood Pressure is hosted by Arthur Ashe, legendary tennis great and heart attack victim. This video will help you learn how heredity and life-style affect your blood pressure, how to understand the disease clearly, and, most importantly, how to live with high blood pressure.

Lower Your Cholesterol Now! is an upbeat, informative, and practical video. Dietician Leni Reed provides clear answers and dozens of tips on how to make wise nutritional choices to lower calories, saturated fat, and cholesterol in your diet. This video is ideal for either self-instruction or group programs.

Stanford Health and Exercise Program brings together renowned fitness specialists and world-class athletes to introduce the concepts and practical tools presented in the accompanying handbook, *The Stanford Health and Exercise Handbook*. Like the book, the video makes an ideal guide for your ongoing fitness efforts at home. Sections feature eight prime benefits of exercise, determining your basic level of fitness, the actual Stanford Workout program, three low-impact aerobic workouts, and more.

Swing into Shape is a low-intensity nonaerobic exercise video for the aging population. It offers the benefits of exercise including the improvement of muscle tone, strength, and flexibility. The three 26-minute routines are designed to acknowledge the physical limitations of this population. Designed by Betsy Bork, physical therapist.

The next five videos are available from Nutrition Counseling and Education Services (NC&ES),

P.O. Box 3018, Olathe, KS 66062-3018. Write for prices and ordering information, or call (913) 782-8230. The following toll-free number is for placing orders only: (800) 445-5653. All videos in VHS format only.

Any Body Can Sit and Be Fit was commissioned by the Illinois State Medical Auxiliary for use in nursing homes by the wheelchair-bound or other individuals who find it difficult to stand and do exercise. Flexibility is improved by following the exercises in this 20-minute video.

Fitness Walking Program teaches you how to set up your own walking program, provides the music to walk by, and teaches you how to do warm-up and cool-down exercises. An 80-page booklet is provided.

Supermarket Savvy Tour Video, by Leni Reed, is an acclaimed video that takes you on a tour through a supermarket. Reed guides you through the aisles, while instructing you in the art of label-reading. Learn how to make informed, healthier choices of food and how to sort out the important information from the mumbo-jumbo. A must if you are concerned about cholesterol and fat in your diet.

Thin Dining is the video to watch to learn how to prescreen restaurants, order assertively, and eat well in ethnic restaurants while minimizing calories. You'll also learn "damage control" for fast-food restaurants, and how to select airline meals.

Warming Up: The Gentle Exercise Videotape for Formerly Inactive People. This program is designed for all people who want to start, or get back to, enjoying regular exercise for fun, healing, and health. Also valuable to people who are overweight.

GOVERNMENT, CONSUMER, AND ADVOCACY GROUPS

American Council of Science and Health (ACSH), 1995 Broadway, 16th Floor, New York, NY 10023, (212) 362-7044

The purpose of this organization is to provide consumers with scientifically balanced evaluations of food, chemicals, the environment, and human health. Council personnel participate in government regulatory proceedings, public debates, and other forums, and regularly write for professional and scientific journals, popular magazines, and newspaper columns. The council also holds national press conferences and produces a self-syndicated series of health updates for radio. It provides 24-hour computer on-line articles featuring commentary, press releases, and questions and answers on health topics. Publishes brochures and pamphlets on numerous health topics and research reports on public health and environmental issues.

American Dietetic Association (ADA), 216 West Jackson Boulevard, Suite 800, Chicago, IL, 60606-6995, (800) 877-1600

The ADA is the major professional organization for the dietetic profession. With over 40,000 members, the ADA is the premiere authoritative source for information related to foods and nutrition.

American Health Foundation (AHF), 320 East 43rd Street, New York, NY 10017, (212) 953-1900

Devoted to promoting preventive medicine, emphasizing four major fields: research (nutrition, environmental carcinogenesis, molecular biology, experimental pathology, and epidemiology); clinical research and services for adults and children (through mini-screening and intervention); public health action (educating laypeople and medical personnel in the principles of preventive medicine); and health economics research (investigating the costs of disease and comparing them with the costs of preventive approaches). Publishes *Health Letter*, bimonthly.

American Heart Association (AHA), 7320 Greenville Avenue, Dallas, TX 75231, (214) 373-6300

The AHA supports research, education, and community service programs with the goal of reducing premature death and disability from stroke and cardiovascular disease. It also publishes several books and periodicals related to healthy heart management.

Bureau Of Health Education (BHE), 1300 Cliffs Road, Building 14, Atlanta, GA 30333, (404) 329-3235

Provides leadership and program direction for the prevention of disease, disability, premature death, and undesirable and unnecessary health problems through health education. Inquiries on health education can be directed to BHE.

National Association of Anorexia Nervosa and Associated Disorders (ANAD), Box 7, Highland Park, IL 60035, (312) 831-3438

Offers assistance to anorexics, bulimics, their families, and others interested in the problems of anorexia nervosa and bulimia. Maintains chapters in 45 states. Seeks better understanding of and prevention and cures for these eating disorders. Educates the public and health professionals on these illnesses and their treatments. Acts as a resource center, compiling and providing information. Works to end discrimination, and fights against the use of misleading advertising and the production, marketing, and distribution of dangerous diet aids.

The Obesity Foundation (TOF), 5600 South Quebec, Suite 160-D, Englewood, CO 80111

Philanthropic organization that seeks to control, and ultimately cure, the disease of obesity. Provides educational courses and materials for health-care professionals and the public on issues pertaining to obesity and weight-loss methods. Sponsors research programs including research on the effects of dietary zinc supplementation in weight control. The foundation plans to operate a toll-free information line, encourage health insurance plans to cover obesity treatment, and improve communication between physicians and the public. Publishes pamphlets and *Trim and Fit,* quarterly.

President's Council On Physical Fitness And Sports, Washington, DC 20201, (202) 755-7478

The council conducts a public service advertising program and cooperates with governmental and private groups to promote the development of physical fitness leadership, facilities, and programs. Produces educational materials on exercise, school physical education programs, and sports and physical fitness for youths, adults, and the elderly.

Index

Page 2 Copyright © March 2, 1987, U.S. News & World Report. Page 6 Table 1.1 Reprinted courtesy of the Metropolitan Life Insurance Company. Page 7 Copyright © 1988/89 by The New York Times Company. Reprinted by permission. Page 10 Copyright © 1988/89 by The New York Times Company. Reprinted by permission. Page 20 Table 1.2 Reprinted courtesy of the Metropolitan Life Insurance Company. Page 29 Copyright © 1988 Time Warner Inc. Reprinted by permission. Page 31 From *Tufts University Diet & Nutrition Letter,* November 1987, page 1. Reprinted by permission. Page 35 Copyright © 1988/89 by The New York Times Company. Reprinted by permission. Page 39 Figure 2.4 *The American Medical Association Family Medical Guide* by the American Medical Association. Copyright © 1982 by the American Medical Association. Reprinted by permission

of Random House, Inc. Page 40 Reprinted with permission from Consumers' Research Magazine, Washington, D.C. Page 46 Courtesy of *Vogue.* Copyright © 1988 by the Conde Nast Publications Inc. Page 56 Copyright © 1988/89 by The New York Times Company. Reprinted by permission. Page 60 Copyright © 1988/89 by The New York Times Company. Reprinted by permission. Page 65 Table 3.1 Copyright © 1990 by Consumers Union of United States, Inc., Mount Vernon, NY 10553. Excerpted by permission from *Consumer Reports Health Letter,* February 1990. Page 75 Reprinted with permission from *Healthline.* Page 84 From *Tufts University Diet & Nutrition Letter,* May 1990, page 1. Reprinted by permission. Page 87 Reprinted by permission from *Changing Times,* The Kiplinger Magazine, April 1989. Copyright © 1989 by The Kiplinger Washington Editors, Inc.

Page 90 Reprinted with permission of American Health Publishing Company, Dallas, Texas. K. D. Brownell, "The Dieting Readiness Test." *The Weight Control Digest,* 1990, 1:6-8. Page 96 Reprinted by permission from page 210 of *Nutrition: An Applied Science* by Patsy Bostick-Reed. Copyright © 1980 by West Publishing Company. All rights reserved. Page 109 By Patricia Long. Reprinted from *In Health.* Copyright © 1989. Page 114 *American Health Magazine,* Copyright © 1988, by Kevin Cobb. Page 116 Table 6.1 Copyright © by Williams and Wilkins, 1989. Page 117 Table 6.2 Copyright © by Williams and Wilkins, 1989. Page 119 Table 6.3 Copyright © by Williams and Wilkins, 1989. Page 120 Copyright © 1988/89 by The New York Times Company. Reprinted by permission. Page 125 Reprinted courtesy of *Healthline.*